Understanding & Healing Hypothyroid (Hashimotos)

Take charge of your health with knowledge, tools & lifestyle practices to heal auto-immune hypo-thyroid (Hashimoto's)

By Deepti Kulkarni Bakshi

This book is dedicated to my husband Sanket Bakshi & my daughter Arusha without whom my journey towards healing my thyroid would have never started. Their support and encouragement to share my knowledge and experiences is why I could complete this book.

Table of Contents

Introduction

It was almost after ten years of living with Hashimoto's that I finally discovered how to turn back its progression. Ten years of highly unpredictable health are morally destructing. Although I have seen hypo-thyroid symptoms since 2004, it took me over two years till I was finally diagnosed with "hypo-thyroidism" in 2006. Another 7 years of living with the symptoms while I was still on the medication. Disappointed by the lack of support and options from the conventional medicine doctors, finally in 2012, my husband started looking into the medical science himself. In two years, by 2014, he on-boarded me on the research that he had found and I had already started reversing my disease. The symptoms were gone, my blood tests improved, my dosage for medication decreased, blood glucose response improved and I got totally off my blood sugar medication. After this life changing experience, as I opened up and started talking more and more to people about my condition, I realized that I was not alone. That is when I decided to share my journey, my experiences and the learnings with all the people out there.

At the time when I was diagnosed back in 2004, the doctor put me on one pill that I was to take throughout the rest of my life. Most of you with an existing thyroid condition might already be aware of this pill – the levothyroxine. The solution sounded much simple, until we realized that it was just introducing the synthetic thyroid hormone in effort to keep my thyroid levels stable. This still did not help me with most of my symptoms. Nor did it cure the actual condition. The solution was to just manage my thyroid hormone levels on a regular basis.

As the days passed, my symptoms started getting worse. Fatigue and hair loss was a regular thing. With it, also came depression and anxiety. All typical hypo-thyroid symptoms like mood-swings, irregular & painful menstrual periods, dry skin, brain fog were there with me almost all the time. What's worse is that it was not just the hypo-thyroid symptoms for me. There was always an occasional bout of symptoms that resembled more like "hyper" thyroid rather than hypo. Those were the times when I was super energetic all day, shed weight within hours, had a racing heart throughout the night. This was probably the most intriguing thing about my condition. Although the doctors could easily explain that I was hypo-thyroid, these occasional bouts of "hyper" symptoms were completely un-explainable.

Over a period of next 4 years after my diagnosis, the doctor increased my thyroid hormone dosage from 25 mcg to 100 mcg and still the symptoms continued. I kept gaining weight during this period. Four years into the disease progression, I was working with some of the doctors at University of California (UC Davis). During this time, the doctors ran a thyroid anti-body panel on me and that's when I discovered that my hypothyroidism was actually being caused by an auto-immune condition. I also discovered that this was what was called – Hashimotos.

At this time, we had changed more than 6 doctors in the hope of healing the condition. Since my thyroid condition was associated with the polycystic ovarian syndrome (PCOS), I was also having trouble conceiving and starting a family. Later, I learnt that PCOS is very frequently associated with hypo-thyroidism in women – especially when there are also blood sugar imbalances. Also, as you will see further in the book, it is very common for thyroid and diabetes to be hand in hand for many of us. The doctors at UC Davis, put me on blood sugar controlling drug – Metformin and suggested some lifestyle changes. With the help of that, I was finally able to conceive in 2009. Given my history with blood glucose imbalances, during my pregnancy, I also had gestational diabetes. A condition due to which my pregnancy was at high-risk during the entire tenure. My diet was limited to boiled vegetables. No rice, no sugar and shots of insulin before each meal. With all that, I think I am really lucky that in May of 2010, I delivered a beautiful and healthy baby daughter – Arusha.

Post pregnancy, I was back to the escalating weight and increasing thyroid hormone dosage. At the peak of it, I was at 125 mcg and still suffering from major fatigue and weight gain problems. It was then that we decided to do something about it ourselves and not rely on the doctors to solve our problems. The last two years however have been really significant. Since that is when we really started getting much deeper into the working of Hashimoto's. At this time, nor I am just able to get a stable hormonal state, but I have also successfully started a reversal of my thyroid dosage which has twice been lowered since then. This happened after we started exploring the science and medicine books ourselves instead of the doctor visits.

Some two years ago, the night time reading for my husband changed from novels and light reading to reading medical research papers and articles that explained the intricate way hormones worked in our body. The mighty powers of the Internet helped him navigate the way through cryptic medical terms and text and after spending a good six months at it, he was finally able to start reading through medical research papers without a need for an interpreter.

The Internet has democratized information and this is exactly what helped us out of my condition. There are several credible sources of such medical research information that are now accessible to everyone.

- The National Center of Biotechnology Information at the US National Library of Medicine has developed and maintained PubMed. PubMed is a free resource and an excellent start for accessing latest and cutting edge medical research papers and articles. It covers the fields of biomedicine, life sciences, behavioral sciences, chemical sciences and bio-engineering.
- The Microsoft Academic Search project also allows you to easily access articles in medical and scientific journals and provides a solid repository for digging into specific research material in Biology and Medicine. This is another great resource recommended.
- Government and Medical agencies such as the FDA (Food and Drug Administration), American Heart Association (AHA), and American Diabetes Association (ADA) publishes a lot of information on their websites that is easily accessible to common person.

The democratization of access to medical research information allowed by these sources was one of the key things that have enabled me unravel the mysterious world of medicine and get to some of the key answers that we were looking for over the last decade. Pouring over literally hundreds of such cutting edge research papers, articles and alternate medicine strategies, we were able to start putting together pieces of information in meaningful sense. The conversations with the doctors vastly improved once I had an understanding of some of the fundamental concepts and access to the latest information. What I also discovered is that we are today experiencing such complicated health conditions mostly because of the deviations from good food and lifestyle today. In my case, all it took was a real serious look at the diet and lifestyle aspects to start the reversal.

My purpose for writing this book was to spread the information that I had learnt in last two years and provide other Hashimoto's patients with tools that they can use to take charge of their own health. More importantly to provide them with a hope of living a better life for remaining of the years. This book is by no means meant to be a prescriptive guidance for Hashimoto's patients. However, it does discuss a few strategies that worked for me to correct my condition. These are also the strategies learnt from various different branches of medicine and how they help cure hormonal imbalances. It also aims at providing knowledge as a valuable tool so that the Hashimoto's patients are able to better understand their condition and take meaningful steps towards making it better.

I am not an author of the best-selling novel. Nor am I a doctor. So obviously, this book does not come with any marketing fluff or a climax building approach. There is no magic diet that I plan to introduce here. I understand that each of us are already occupied with lots of different things throughout the day. If you are reading a book about thyroid, you will get just that – the information. Which is also why the book is short and not a 400 page novel. When you start reading this book, I try to get to the point, deliver the information and get out of it.

The concepts & strategies discussed in this book are not new. As you may see in some of the later chapters, the concepts are around in the medical research world since more than a decade at this time. Unfortunately, we do not see these being implemented by endocrinologists to help the Hashimoto's patients. I have heard that there are also several registered medical practitioners who are trying these out successfully. However, such examples are still far from the main stream and are far and few between. It is probably the disconnection between medical research world and the practical physician's world that we are dealing with.

This book is intended for any person suffering from Hashimoto's or who just wants to generally understand this condition better. It aims to provide knowledge about the disease and about how it can be healed by using some of the body's innate healing capabilities. I tried to keep this book simple, crisp and precise enough so that it can be read and understood by anyone who does not have much understanding about biology or medicine. The biological processes and terms are explained in simple words and diagrams that can be easily grasped by a common person. In a nutshell, this book is a simplified version of all the knowledge that I gained about Hashimoto's as a common person with no medical background. I intend to help simplify your journey if you wish to take the same path.

It is said that most of the cutting edge research does not make it to the medical curriculum several years after it is released. I know a lot of statistics get made up on the Internet. So it is pointless to argue if this is a true statistic or not. But from what we see from the research, it does seem to indicate some relevance to this number. A good example of this is a 1998 research study that had shown a strong link between Auto-immune thyroid diseases and gluten sensitivity. Almost 15 years later, the doctors still (almost) never test for gluten sensitivity for thyroid patients.

| Research Bits

Check it out for yourself. The study titled **"Autoimmune thyroid diseases and coeliac disease"** was published in Nov 1998 in the European Journal of Gastroenterology & Hepatology by Department of Internal Medicine of Universita' di Torino in Italy. The study can be search on Pubmed (www.pubmed.com). It strongly suggests that all the autoimmune thyroid patients be tested for gluten intolerance. [1]

However, as you start delving into this further, these studies provide us with good insights into how the science of medicine is shaping and what the future for our cure will look like. At the same time, when these are about trying out diet and lifestyle changes, it is also much easier to try on oneself without much risk of any side effects or adverse effects of any kind. We definitely do not discuss introducing any additional medication here. Any changes to the medication of course need to be done along with your doctor and not in isolation.

With this book, I also intend to advertise the democratization of medical information. Demonstrate that a non-medical person can have the ability to gain an understanding and appreciation of their own condition and make a positive difference. A difference that most of the doctors are unfortunately not able to offer today due to various different reasons outside the scope of this book. The book intends to make you a savvy Hashimoto's patient. I quote a lot of research articles in this book. For some, it might seem like a case of selective picking of the research. I have seen many people out there making a single point with selective picking of the research. Yes. I did pick the research that I quote here. But then as you would explore, the research is from a variety of different fields, variety of different aspects impacting thyroid and we link it all together with simple common sense and a bit of logic. It's hard for me to believe that research across multiple streams when looked in conjunction with each other can really deliver a distorted picture. But in any case, this is of course my interpretation of the medical research. In the last chapter of this book, I share how I went ahead with reading and understanding this research and piecing it together. This I believe is the single biggest benefit of this book. If you are a nerd like I am, this gives you enough power to take a deep dive and explore your health condition for yourself. Democratization of the information is a powerful tool. A double edge sword in fact that should be used carefully to the best benefit. I would argue for the most that when embarking on your own journey with this information, use this information as a tool to communicate well with the doctor. Most of the suggestions in this book are fairly harmless – just impacting the diet and lifestyle aspects. But this should not disconnect us from the doctor. Especially with the thyroid condition it is of utmost importance that you work along with your doctor with the information provided in this book. Mismanagement with the thyroid can be a life-threatening situation.

The chapters in this book are laid out to provide you a technical understanding of the thyroid mechanisms and auto-immunity. I tried to simplify this technical understanding with simpler words and even simpler images and flowcharts to explain the concepts. Further, the book delves into strategies to better understand the condition with an existing set of medical tools available today and work with the doctor for best results. Lastly, it provides actionable items that were found to helpful based on publicly published research and our own experimentation for a positive change towards healing Hashimoto's and overall health.

Throughout the book, relevant points have "Research Bits" and "Lab Tests" marked that will provide material for further research on your own and help empower you to better understand your specific situation. Each of us have a unique body that will behave and respond slightly differently to the same external stimulus. Hence, these Research bits will provide you with the right information that will allow you to take charge of your own health.

As kids, we have almost always experienced the healing capabilities of the human body. Be it a scratch or a wound or a digestive disorder. We've always seen that given the time and the right nutrition for the body, the body wants to heal itself. It knows how to heal itself – much better than we think. It never wants to be in a broken state. That's a fundamental premise of this book. That's the fundamental understanding that the cutting edge medical research has revealed as well in very near past. As you would see further in this book, the strategies that we talk about here, basically get us to the root cause, help eliminate the underlying triggers of the condition and from there simply help the body heal itself.

Just like us, the human body does not like to be in a broken state.

What does the normal Thyroid function look like?

According to US Department of Health & Human Services, over 4.6 percent of population in United States over the age of 12 suffers from Hypothyroidism[i]. This is as per the statistics in 2009 and cases of Hypothyroidism are rapidly increasing today. The symptoms of hypothyroidism have a strong overlap with overweight and obesity which is also the reason why there are many more cases that are not even diagnosed as several thousands of people struggle with weight gain and low energy levels while going completely undiagnosed of thyroid issues and blame their condition on the ever increasing weight. In any case, when we talk about Hypothyroidism, we are talking about a significantly high number of the population.

The thyroid hormone itself plays a significant role in the functioning of a normal human body. This chapter digs deeper into the scientific understanding of the thyroid & auto immune thyroid conditions such as Hashimoto's. Although it delves a bit deep into the science and might be at times very technical and hence difficult to follow, this understanding is critical for managing and making a positive change to the thyroid disorders.

The Thyroid gland is a part of what is known as the endocrine system in the human body. The endocrine system comprises of multiple organs that secrete some key hormones and control important functions of the body including metabolism, growth and sexual development. The Thyroid gland is responsible for secreting the thyroid hormone. The thyroid hormone helps "activate" the individual cells in the body and allows them to perform their specific functions. Due to this specific function thyroid forms a very crucial part of the endocrine system and directly impacts the metabolic functions when its functioning is disturbed. Recent research has also discovered strong associations with degraded neural functions with an impaired thyroid function.

The gland itself is a butterfly shaped organ, approximately the size of the pinky finger and sitting in front of the neck below the voice box.

Let's take a look at a simplistic model of how the thyroid and its feedback mechanisms work. There is definitely a lot more at play here with intricate reverse feedback mechanisms. However, this will give a good starter for understanding of the processes involved.

The thyroid hormone is actually a collection of multiple different hormones - T4 (thyroxine), T3 (triiodothyronine) & rT3 (Reverse T3). T3 is more active form of the hormone and part of T4 produced by the thyroid gland also gets used to convert to T3. Which is why abnormally low levels or T4 can have a direct impact on T3 as well. It is estimated that the thyroid gland actually secretes approximately 20% of the T3 found in the bloodstream. The rest of circulating T3 or what is known as Free T3 is converted from T4 within the Liver, Kidneys & even the small intestine. The Reverse T3 is also partly generated by the thyroid gland but mostly produced as a by-product of the T4 to t3 conversion process after monitoring the circulating T3 levels in the bloodstream.

The Thyroid gland generates these hormones in response to a specific signal from the pituitary gland. This signal is what is known as the Thyroid stimulating hormone (TSH). As the name suggests, the TSH stimulates the thyroid gland to produce more the thyroid hormone. The pituitary secretion of TSH is in turn controlled by the Thyroid Releasing Hormone (TRH) that is released by the Hypothalamus. The overall process of thyroid hormone production is strictly controlled by tight feedback loops by the hypothalamus-pituitary-thyroid axis by monitoring the free circulating levels of T3, T4 & rT3.

Once the T3 & T4 is available in the bloodstream, it is used by the individual cells in the body to help them perform their functions. Every cell in the human body has specific receptors for the hormones that it needs. In case of the thyroid hormone receptors (TR), the T3 has significantly higher number of receptors on the individual cells than T4. Which is really the reason why T3 is considered to be more active hormone than T4. The metabolic effects of the thyroid hormones are seen when the hormones bind themselves to the specific cell receptor sites and make themselves available for reactions and processes within the cells.

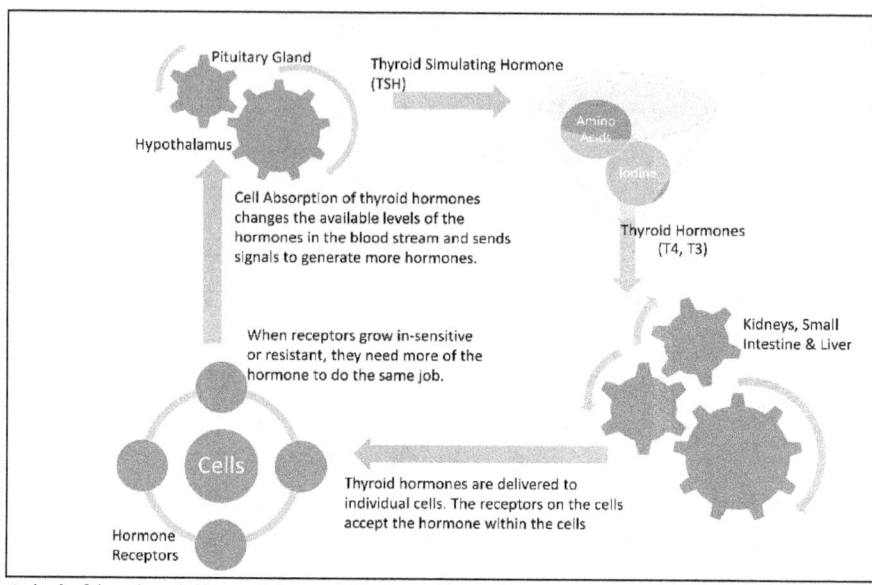

Pituitary Gland

Thyroid Simulating Hormone (TSH)

Hypothalamus

Amino Acids

Iodine

Cell Absorption of thyroid hormones changes the available levels of the hormones in the blood stream and sends signals to generate more hormones.

Thyroid Hormones (T4, T3)

When receptors grow in-sensitive or resistant, they need more of the hormone to do the same job.

Kidneys, Small Intestine & Liver

Cells

Thyroid hormones are delivered to individual cells. The receptors on the cells accept the hormone within the cells

Hormone Receptors

A brief look at thyroid and its feedback mechanism.

Hashimoto's: Hypothyroid & Autoimmunity

We are all aware of the role that immune system plays in protecting the body from external attackers such as viruses. The immune system is body's defense mechanism. Whenever a body is attacked by any external pathogen, the immune system responds countering the attack and ensuring that the body is kept safe.

Typically, the immune system has multiple ways of doing this. In certain cases it can raise the overall inflammation in a particular area of the body or in other cases, it will work by creating precise anti bodies that will target the specific pathogen that attacks the body. In case of the auto-immune diseases, the immune system "thinks" of the organ tissue as an external invader and generates anti-bodies against it. These antibodies are called self-antigens since they are attacking the same body that they are hosted in. Hence, it's really the body's immune system working against a specific tissue in the body. In cases of auto-immune thyroid, it is the thyroid that is under attack by the immune system.

The human body has a number of counter-balancing techniques. Auto-immunity attacks on tissues are a common occurrence within the body. In general cases, the human body generates what is known as Regulatory T-cells (Tregs). The TRegs, are responsible maintaining the tolerance of self-antigens and ensuring that auto-immunity does not kick in.

However, in case of auto-immune thyroid conditions, the specific Tregs responsible for regulating the immune attack on thyroid are dysfunctional and hence the disease progresses. In the absence of normally functioning Tregs, the auto-immune attack gets fuelled by subsequent triggers and the auto-immune condition continues to progress. Recent research has found that the polymorphism or mutation of certain genes can be influencing the TRegs behavior and overall susceptibility of auto-immune thyroid conditions.

In summary, any auto immune thyroid condition (Hashimoto's or Graves) has a strong genetic link. This is combined with certain environmental triggers that trigger the immune system to generate the thyroid antibodies. Subsequently, the auto-immune regulation function breaks down causing it to become a full blown auto-immune condition that can be fuelled by subsequent triggers.

The triggers in such cases can be varied ranging from sustained low grade inflammations, parasite infections, dietary choices, not enough sleep, stress, antibiotics administration, absence of proper 'good bacteria' in the gut, or even trauma caused due to serious events.

While we do see multiple triggers here, the manifestation of the auto-immune disease starts by these triggers impacting the vitality of the small intestine or what is commonly known as the 'gut'. The small intestine, is where most of the food gets processed and assimilated into the bloodstream. The gut is one of the key 'barriers' in our system that separates the food coming in from outside of the system from the internal organs and the bloodstream. In order to achieve this separation while still allowing the assimilation of digested food in the bloodstream, the small intestine has a mesh like lining. In a healthy gut, this lining will allow only finely digested particles of food to escape in the bloodstream. Any un-digested food, which would be a bigger particle in nature, would be carried over to the large intestine and subsequently excreted out of the system.

When some of the triggers discussed above hit, this lining of the gut gets compromised resulting in larger opening through which food particles that are not completely digested can escape into the bloodstream. This compromising of the gut is also sometimes referred to as a "leaky gut". Since these bigger undigested particles are usually not expected in the bloodstream, the immune system kicks in thinking of these as foreign bodies or viruses.

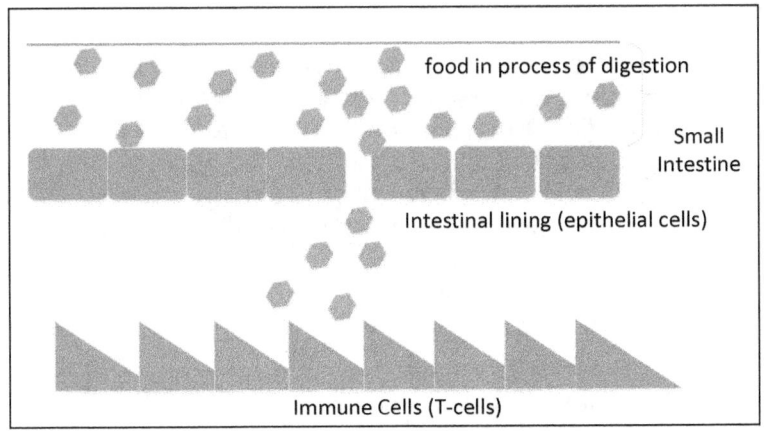

food in process of digestion

Small Intestine

Intestinal lining (epithelial cells)

Immune Cells (T-cells)

In certain cases, the protein structures of such undigested particles can resemble a specific organ tissue of the body itself. Thus, when the immune system prepares an anti-body for such particles, it is in fact also creating an antibody for the organ as well. This phenomenon of the similarity in the molecular structure causing the confusion with the immune system is known as molecular mimicry. In cases of Hashimoto's, the organ tissues that mimic such particles will be the thyroid enzymes. Hence, the antibodies for those are created and thus, the reaction of auto-immunity starts.

▍Research Bits

Shift Work in Teens Linked to Increased Multiple Sclerosis Risk: The National Sleep Foundation discusses the link between disturbances of circadian rhythms and auto-immunity with this article at (http://sleepfoundation.org/)[3]

New diseases derived or associated with the tight junction
This 2007 article in the Archives of Medical Research describes the mechanism of intestinal tight junctions and links several auto-immune conditions (including thyroid disorders) to compromising of such junctions. The most popular being the compromising of the tight junction in the small intestinal. Commonly known as the leaky gut.

Multiple studies have shown lifestyle factors such as sleep pattern disorders, chronic stress, yeast or parasite infections to contribute towards the leaky gut and thus starting the cascade of the auto-immune conditions.

Most of my strategies for managing my thyroid condition have revolved around this understanding of the mechanism. I realized that effectively managing the intestinal permeability while providing good support for my thyroid to resume its own functioning, helped me recover quickly.

Working with the doctor

For many people already diagnosed with an auto-immune thyroid condition, working with the doctor to "manage" the condition is very common and in fact a necessity. This chapter delves into details of understanding how you can use the conventional medicine tools to better understand your condition and help you navigate through remediating it. Working with your doctor is also an integral part of remediation process and should be used as a tool.

The most important thing to understand here is that while we work on remediating the conditions, it is important NOT to discontinue any medication before talking to the doctor. As you follow the diet and lifestyle changes in this book, you will periodically work with your doctor to test and lower the thyroid hormone supplementation as is deemed appropriate by your blood tests. Some of these strategies and ideas for opening up the conversations with the doctors will be discussed further in this chapter.

Throughout this book, we have been talking about various different studies. An important point to note here is that these studies are not just from the conventional medicine. Conventional or Western or allopathic medicine is what most of us are intimately familiar with. However, apart from this, there are also a few other lesser known medicinal practices such as functional medicine, naturopathic medicine, Ayurvedic medicine, Nutritional Science and even the Chinese herbal medicine. Each of these has their own strengths and shortcomings. Throughout my decade long agony and dealing with the conventional western medicine doctors, one thing was evident – that they do not have all the answers that I needed. When my husband and I started looking into the research ourselves, we figured that alternative medicine practices such as functional medicine or Ayurvedic medicine and even nutritional science has already made significant strides in some of the areas where conventional medicine has stopped. The studies and the protocols that I discuss in this book, are a combination of what I learnt from my research in all of these practices.

What I also saw is that when I spoke to the conventional medicine doctors about a lot of these concepts, some of them were not very receptive, the others listened but did not know what to do much after that. For instance, figuring out the autoimmune aspect of thyroid was easy, but the treatment from conventional medicine standpoint, still remained exactly the same. Whereas, functional medicine already has a huge amount of research and success in addressing that. Similarly, Ayurvedic medicine has some proven practices around helping the thyroid gland improve the production of the hormone without external support. Nutritional science has a good deal of research on how to reduce the inflammatory load and provide ample nutrition to the body to aid the healing process.

Nobody can own your health better than yourself. With the differences between different medical practices, I am now a firm believer in not having a primary care physician or an endocrinologist manage by thyroid problems alone. I believe that we need to be able to form a team of doctors that will together help us get to a better state of health. A team that spans across different streams of medicinal practices to get a diverse opinion. As a patient, you own your health and have the onus of orchestrating this team for your best benefit. Each of these team members needs to be open on perspectives and need to understand that this is not about their capabilities or their own ego. It is more about how they can help you achieve your health goals. It takes some time to whet out who you would want on this team. The idea here is not to test the doctors for their knowledge. I don't think we are technically capable of doing that, especially since each of them is of course an expert in their own field. However, the most important factor is the comfort factor that you would have with the doctor as well as the doctor's openness to accepting that he is not the only person you will be interacting with. There might be cases where the doctors can have conflicting opinions and each of them need to be presenting their case to you as the patient so that you can make a decision. End of the day, it is your health. You need to be in charge.

Later parts of this book will help you guide towards the specific diet and lifestyle aspects. But having this team in place will help you monitor the progress and keep making the changes as are required for your individual case. Each individual is different and while the recommendations in here will apply to everyone, having these doctors help you along your journey will help with the specific cases that you might have.

Do note however that the insurance model here in the United States, most often does not cover alternative medicine practices. So it definitely is a significant cost when it comes to assembling the team that we discussed. If that is the concern, I would recommend that you at least make sure that you are following the diet and lifestyle guidelines in this book to a tee. Also, during this time, make sure that you are completely comfortable having a deeper conversation with your endocrinologist. Make sure that you have access to the blood tests that we discuss further to help you monitor your progress along the way. Make sure that he understands the diet and lifestyle choices that you are making and supports those. Having a solid support from your doctor will go a long way in making your healing journey a lot more comfortable.

The Thyroid Management Protocol

If you are already diagnosed with Hypothyroidism, you might've already had some blood tests done for the diagnosis. In most of the cases, chances are that you've seen the TSH value go through the roof which is why you were put on the thyroid pills. The National Endocrine and Metabolic Diseases Information Service (NEMDIS) suggest that hypothyroidism be treated with synthetic thyroxine. This is a medication that is identical to T4 that we discussed in one of the previous chapters. The dosage of this medication depends on several factors including age, weight and severity of hypothyroidism and presence of any other health conditions or administration of other drugs that may impact the body's ability to use this synthetic hormone.

However, the only marker from the blood test that is used to determine the 'severity' of the disease is the TSH. The TSH values are usually tested regularly and if needed the dosage is adjusted accordingly. This works well for most of the patients, till the time they take the thyroid pill each day.

▌Research Bits

Hypothyroidism Treatment: The National Endocrine and Metabolic Diseases Information Service (NEMDIS) discusses hypothyroidism and its treatments on their website at (http://endocrine.niddk.nih.gov)[4]

This management protocol looks good on the face of it. This is also what I followed for over a decade before we got access to more information leading to some important questions.

The overall process of generating and metabolizing the thyroid hormones in the body is a complex system based on several feedback loops. Looking at it objectively, we can see that there are multiple points of failure in the system –

- The pituitary gland or the hypothalamus can be malfunctioning due to which the TSH signals cannot be generated appropriately for the thyroid gland to produce the thyroid hormone.
- The Thyroid gland can itself be dysfunctional and not be generating enough T4 / T3

- The thyroid gland might not be getting enough raw material (probably Iodine deficiency) to generate the hormones
- Once the T4 is generated, the T4 might not be getting converted to T3 properly in the liver or other organs.
- The Thyroid hormone receptors on the cells might be resistant to the thyroid hormone, hence they need more of it. (Similar to insulin resistance in diabetes)
- The functioning of the thyroid gland might be hindered due to constant attacks from the immune system and hence it is not able to generate enough hormone (auto-immune attack).

At any given time, one or more of these can be true in a hypothyroidism patient. Each of these conditions will also result in an elevated TSH value thus making it completely impossible to determine the underlying cause of high TSH when looking at the blood tests reports. Depending on which of these mechanisms is broken, it might be completely possible to reverse the disease. For instance, less Iodine intake can cause lower thyroid production and that can be easily fixed by increasing the amount of Iodine (although with some other considerations). Or the conversion of T4 to T3 in the liver might be impacted because the liver is already overwhelmed with cleaning multiple toxins in the body. Hence a medically supervised detoxification might be able to resolve the issues there.

Several recent studies have also indicated correlations between the common metabolic disorders such as Diabetes and thyroid dysfunctions. The verdict however is not yet out if thyroid disorders cause the metabolic disorders or vis-a-versa. However, the correlation sure exists.

In any case, as can be seen from these multiple factors, the usual protocol of monitoring only TSH values falls woefully short of understand the underlying cause of the problem and definitely needs further attention.

This book focuses specifically on the auto-immune thyroid conditions that are probably the most prevalent of the conditions. Hence, one of the very first steps will be to understand if what you have is an auto-immune condition. We discussed about the auto-immunity and thyroid in the earlier chapter and I would definitely suggest that you go through that to better understand the context of what auto-immune thyroid conditions mean. Auto-immunity is one of the most common causes of hypothyroidism and can be easily found out by a readily available blood test.

▎Lab Tests

The following blood tests are the most common ones used to identify if the hypothyroid is due to an auto-immune condition.

Thyroid Peroxidase (TPO) Antibody – TPOAb
This test checks for the *"Thyroid Peroxidase (TPO) Antibody"*. The TPO is a gene that helps the body generate an enzyme called thyroid peroxidase. This enzyme is crucial for the thyroid gland to generate the thyroid hormone. The TPO antibodies usually target the TPO enzymes. With the enzymes not being available for the chemical reaction, the thyroid gland is not able to generate the hormones in required quantities. Presence of TPOAb outside the usual limits indicate an auto-immune condition.

Thyroglobulin Antibody (TgAb)

This test checks for the antibodies to thyroglobulin. These anti-bodies can be found after damage or trauma to the thyroid gland. These anti-bodies target thyroglobulin – a protein that is used by the thyroid gland to create thyroid hormones. These anti-bodies are also known to cause damage to the thyroid gland itself making the healing process more time-consuming. Over 90% of cases with TPOAb also have elevated levels TgAb.

In certain cases, patients having hypothyroidism symptoms may have a TSH in normal range but can have elevated presence of anti-bodies. This condition simply means that the auto-immunity has kicked in but has not impacted enough to cause any imbalances in the thyroid hormones and their associated feedback loops. In such conditions as well, it is highly recommended that appropriate steps be taken for controlling the auto-immunity before it triggers in full-blown hypothyroid condition.

Often times than not, when I talk to other people with such results, or even an abnormal TSH results, their endocrinologists usually do not suggest these blood tests. This is usually because from their perspective, the treatment does not change even if the disease is auto-immune. However, as a patient, you would be able to push further because you want to better understand your own condition.

However, once the tests determine that the hypo-thyroid issues are due to auto-immune condition, the next logical step is to understand what is causing the immune reaction and help pacify the trigger so that the natural production of the hormone can continue.

We already discussed how the cause of the auto-immune disease can be multi-factorial. Various issues such as food sensitivities, sleep, stress etc. can be playing a role in the auto-immunity triggers. These also result in a compromised intestinal lining that further fuels the condition. Given this, it is but obvious that the approach to address these triggers need to be multi-faceted as well.

Let us take a look at some of the most common triggers for auto-immunity and how to test for those. Once the causes are known, the specific diet and lifestyle strategies outlined in the subsequent chapters can be easily applied to devise a plan for your own.

Food Sensitivities

In today's world, the "leaky-gut" or a compromised intestinal barrier is a very common issue. Given the amount of toxins that the body is subjected to through food, water, air & all the other things around us makes us high likely to have a compromised gut lining. The manifestation of auto-immunity is hence a matter of genetic chance. If the body is sensitive to any of the food being eaten, it is very likely to cause an immune flare-up.

To understand the concept of sensitivity, food sensitivities can be thought of as low grade allergies. An allergy however would show an immediate flare-up of the immune system. Sensitivities on the other hand, trigger a low grade inflammation in the body that does not show up as an allergic reaction. However, continuously subjecting the body to the sensitive foods keep a low grade immune flare-up running in the system. This greatly stresses the immune system due to the continuous work involved and does not allow the body to heal the intestine. In most of the cases, it takes several years or even decades for the effects of these sensitivities to manifest into full blown auto-immune conditions. When such conditions occur, it becomes very hard to point these back to the food sensitivities or the compromised intestinal lining because of the time taken for the issues to manifest. Direct co-relation is many times impossible unless we start eliminating the problematic foods.

Gluten has been proved to be the key auto-immunity trigger in almost all the auto-immunity conditions today. Dr. William Davis discusses this in his book "Wheat Belly" and attributes the increase in gluten related food sensitivities today to rampant hybridization of wheat that was done to increase the yield.

Hence, Gluten needs to be completely off the list when it comes to resolving auto-immunity issues.

Gluten sensitivity is a relatively newer concept for mainstream gastroenterology medicine. It's probably even a more remote concept for other streams of medicine such as endocrinology. More than a year ago, when I discussed the gluten sensitivity with my endocrinologist, he readily presented me with a blood test for celiac. Celiac is an intestinal condition that is characterized by almost an allergy response by the body towards gluten. By contrast, gluten sensitivity lies under the covers and does not usually provide immediate visible symptoms. Hence, as expected, my tests for celiac were completely normal and I was told that there are absolutely no issues for my body with gluten. For most of the thyroid patients, the gluten sensitivity never blows up into a full blown celiac disease (gluten allergy) and hence is never really seen on the celiac blood test.

Unfortunately, there is no agreed upon standard for testing gluten sensitivity. Eliminating gluten from the diet & observing the effects is probably one of the best tests for sensitivity. However, given our strong psychological association with the foods, the blood tests sometimes give a much needed morale boost to eliminate gluten. When I first heard about thyroid and gluten connection, that's exactly what I needed – a morale boost to give up gluten. As a person so closely associated with Indian food, roti or the flatbread was almost a staple food and the thought of giving it up was not very pleasant. Giving up gluten was probably the hardest thing that I had to face in last two years. Not surprisingly as well when you see that research in nutritional science has observed gluten and casein to produce opioid like activity in the brain. Thus almost causing an addiction. Studies have observed autistic patients and found significant behavior changes when introduced to gluten.

The Cyrex labs test discussed below is available in the US and was the test that we used to determine the food sensitivities. In our experience, this test provided a fairly good indication of the sensitivities.

In any case, given number of compelling evidences against gluten and thyroid, gluten must be ticked off the foods in any case.

Research Bits

The Department of Medicine at University of Alberta (Canada) published an article in October 2006 that is now available on Pubmed.com.

The article is titled – **Alterations in Intestinal Permeability.** This article discusses the causes for intestinal permeability. It also explores the link between intestinal permeability and auto-immunity in significant details. [5]

The Indian Journal of Medical Research published an article in Nov 2013 that discusses the role of gut in autoimmunity. The article is titled – **Bugs & Us: The role of gut in auto-immunity.** [6]

A 2012 research conducted in Brazil on developmental disorders discusses the opioid like activity in the brain caused due to gluten and casein. This study can be found on pubmed titled – **Intestinal permeability and nutritional status in developmental disorders.**

Lab Tests

In the US, Cyrex Labs (www.cyrexlabs.com) provide an array of tests to determine common food sensitivities.

Gluten-Associated Cross-Reactive Foods and Food Sensitivity
This test checks the blood sample for sensitivity to gluten and certain other cross-reacting foods. Cross reacting foods are basically all the foods which the immune system can potentially mistake for gluten – causing a similar flare up as eating gluten. It checks for foods such as –

- Milk
- Chocolate
- Yeast
- Coffee
- Sesame
- Other grains (Buckwheat, Oats, Millet, Sorghum)
- Tapioca

- Teff
- Soy
- Eggs
- Corn
- Rice
- Potato
- Amaranth
- Hemp

Not to say that this is an exhaustive list, but it is a good starting point to address the food sensitivities.

The Cyrex labs blood test discussed here is definitely an expensive one. As discussed above an alternative, and probably a more definitive way to determine food sensitivities can be simply removing some of the commonly sensitive foods from the diet. In his book, "Why do I still have Thyroid Symptoms", Dr. Datis Kharrazian calls this approach as the provocation diet. Wherein, you provoke the body to show up a food sensitivity response. A similar approach is also advocated by Tom Malterre who terms this as Elimination diet.

The provocation or elimination diet works by eliminating most commonly sensitive foods for a period of time, allowing the gut to heal itself during that time and then finally re-introducing each of the foods one by one to understand the body's response to the foods. The provocation diet also helps you get a lot more in tune with the body and provides a deeper realization of how food impacts the body in several different ways.

The provocation diet would require that the following very commonly sensitive foods are taken completely off the diet for a period of at least 3 weeks.

- Grains (Not just gluten, but all grains)
- Sugar
- Dairy
- Egg
- Soy
- Corn
- Alcohol

While these foods are eliminated the focus will be given on nutrient dense vegetables, specifically green leafy vegetables that will help provide a substantial level of nutrients to nourish and heal the body while the sensitive foods are off the list. Meat, especially fatty cuts and organ meats are also significantly nutrient dense and will be included during this time.

At the end of 3 weeks, introduce one food at time from the previously eliminated list. The foods should be introduced one at a time with at least 3-5 days between the introductions of two different foods. After introducing each food, carefully observe its impact on the body – how does your skin react? Do you feel tired or lethargic? Do you have any significant changes in bowel movements? Any adverse reaction suggests that the body is sensitive to that food and that food should hence be eliminated from the diet at least for next few months. The same food can be introduced at a later time and the effect on the body can be similarly observed.

However, during this process, gluten should be completely eliminated. Due to the massive hybridization of the grains containing gluten and their processing, gluten containing grains is almost a special food that should strictly be avoided in today's world.

40

In certain cases, people have had auto-immune flare up due to Soy as well. If the tests or the provocation diet reflects this, Soy needs to be avoided very similar to gluten.

Stress

Most of us are intimately familiar with a stressful lifestyle today. External pressures including work, social & financial commitments to the least add a great deal of stress towards the body. Stress however, is not just restricted to these visible aspects in life. The body undergoes stress in a number of different ways – some of which we take so much for granted. For instance, food sensitivities discussed earlier in this chapter, cause a significant stress for the immune system. Disturbances in circadian rhythm (lack of sleep or irregular sleep) causes significant hormonal changes, thus inducing internal stress in the body.

Cortisol is known as the stress hormone in the body. It is one of the key hormones that the body uses for wakefulness and alertness. During stressful situations, the body reacts by producing more cortisol. Although occasional bursts of cortisol are healthy for the body and promote increased memory, immunity and similar benefits, constant elevation of this hormones is a key indicator of chronic stress.

A recent study done in Belgium, concludes that acute psychological stress and even elevated cortisol levels results in intestinal permeability in humans. Chronic stress, thus causes a significant impact on the intestinal permeability by not allowing it to heal.

Another article published by John Hopkins School of Medicine, also relates stress to the overall sensitivity of the thyroid receptors on the cells. As we already saw in the earlier chapters, a decreased sensitivity of the receptors, eventually means that more thyroid hormone is needed for the same job, thus resulting in elevated levels of TSH to simulate hormone production.

Stress is thus a double whammy that not just promotes auto-immune conditions for thyroid disorders but also lowers the sensitivity of the receptors, hence causing the thyroid gland to have to work harder for fulfilling the needs of the body.

▎Research Bits

The University of Leuven, Belgium published a research in October 2013 that discusses how stress was found to be linked with intestinal permeability. The research titled **"Psychological stress and corticotropin-releasing hormone increase intestinal permeability in humans by a mast cell-dependent mechanism"** can be found on Pubmed.

Research from John Hopkins Medical School titled **"Chemokine orchestration of autoimmune thyroiditis"** discusses how Chemokines can cause auto-immunity especially related to thyroid. The Chemokines are protein based components typically found to play a role in managing inflammation in the body.

The level of cortisol can be determined by either a blood test or a saliva test. However, given that amount of stressors that are around us today, de-stressing is definitely one of the key strategies for any healing in the body.

> **▌ Lab Tests**
>
> Some of the major labs in the US provide the Adrenal Stress Tests that use either saliva, urine or blood specimen to determine Cortisol and various other stress parameters.

Sleep

As one of the species on the earth, the human body is intricately connected with the cycles of nature. The most commonly known cycle of nature is of course the day and night cycle that we see each day. We've all heard about our own biological clock. In a normal circumstance, this clock would've been attuned to the typical day and night differences of light, temperature and the natural sounds. The fancy medical name for this biological clock is the "Circadian Rhythm".

The circadian rhythms are not just the sleep and wake-up patterns of the body. They are intricately linked with various hormone responses in the body. Rather the hormone responses are what causes the predictable sleep cycles. There is an interlaced play of these hormones when it connects to circadian rhythms. Understanding this play also plays an important part in diet and lifestyle regulation since it allows better enhancement of the sleep patterns.

The research around sleep is increasing each day and we are getting to know various ways in which sleep helps the body. A sound sleep helps the body to refresh, rewire and heal. There are an astounding number of processes that take place in the body when we are asleep and science is just finding that what we know might not even be the tip of the iceberg.

Back in 2009, the International Reviews of Immunology Journal published an article (titled: Circadian Rhythm and the Immune Response: A Review) that explored the relationship between Circadian Rhythms and Auto-immunity. Sleep research has also been shown to aid regeneration of regulatory T-cells (Tregs). In the earlier chapters we discussed how the Tregs play a significant role in development of auto-immunity. From these and more of similar studies, we understand that sleep plays a very important role in hormonal regulation, auto-immunity, neuro-degeneration and several other conditions.

▌Lab Tests

Several major labs perform melatonin assessments using saliva samples. The tests can determine the melatonin rhythms (directly linked to circadian rhythms) & secretion patterns. These can be ordered by tests such as **"Comprehensive Melatonin Profile"** or **"Melatonin Rhythms"**.

Although the lab tests discussed below help understand Melatonin issues, getting these from the conventional medical practitioners would sometimes be a challenge since these are usually used for analysis of neurological issues. Again when it comes to testing, the sleep issues are better "felt" than tested. Here are some of the questions that you can ask yourself to determine if you have issues with quality of sleep –

- Do you spend lot of time in the bed before finally sleeping?
- Do you wake up once or multiple times at night?

- Once awake in the night, do you have trouble sleeping again?
- When waking up in the morning, do you still feel sleepy or groggy?

If any of these symptoms are present for extended duration of time (for continuous few weeks or more), there is a definite disruption in the circadian rhythms and that must be fixed before it further cascades to an impact on the immune system.

Research Bits

The link between circadian rhythms and auto-immunity is discussed in article titled "**Circadian Rhythm and the Immune Response: A Review**". The article was published in International Reviews of Immunology Journal.

The 2010 study titled "**Sleep, Immunity and Circadian Clocks: A Mechanist Model**" discusses how sleep impacts the immune system. The study is published by The University of Luebeck, Germany and can be searched on Microsoft Academic Search.

Vitamin D deficiency

Another most common factor observed is the Vitamin D deficiency. In my case, when we first started to look at the Vitamin D levels, they were down at 16 ng/mL. The normal reference range usually starts at 20 or 25 ng/ml. So I was a lot lower even from the minimum required range.

Now Vitamin D is an interesting Vitamin. If we look at the Vitamin D studies relating the auto-immunity, we see that in almost all the cases, Vitamin D deficiency is seen to be a pre-cursor for not just auto-immune conditions but also to other serious conditions such as Diabetes, Tuberculosis and even Multiple-Sclerosis. The Journal of Allergy and Clinical Immunology has also published a hypothesis that links Vitamin D with food allergies. It takes part in a vast array of metabolic processes within the body and that makes it much more significant than most of the other Vitamins out there.

▎Research Bits

A 2010 study out of Belgium discusses how Vitamin D impacts the immune system and contributes to auto-immunity. This study is title **"Vitamin D: modulator of the immune system"**. This is further explored in another Dec 2014 study from Australia titled **"Vitamin D & Immunity"** and an article from American Journal of Clinical Nutrition titled **"Sunlight and vitamin D for bone health and prevention of autoimmune diseases, cancers, and cardiovascular disease."** Another study out of China in Sep 2014 find correlation between Vitamin D deficiency and oxidative stress in children. This is titled **"Vitamin D status and its association with adiposity and oxidative stress in schoolchildren"**.
All of these studies can be searched on pubmed database.

We discussed intestinal permeability as an initiating mechanism for auto-immunity in the earlier chapters and Vitamin D deficiency also plays a very significant role in that.

Studies have shown that Vitamin D deficiency leads to increased susceptibility to intestinal permeability hence contributing directly to auto-immunity. Recent studies also demonstrate that Vitamin D deficiencies introduce immune dysfunctions. Sometime also making the immune system hyper-active. Specifically in auto-immune conditions, when the immune system is actually attacking your own tissue, a hyper-active immune system just means more damage and a worsened disease condition. Lastly, such deficiencies are also shown to cause significant increase in oxidative stress, thus triggering the body's stress mechanisms and taking us further down the spiral.

When my Vitamin D levels were tested and found to be low, I was put on Vitamin D supplementation of 50000 IU per week. To give a perspective, the daily recommended value is 400 IU. Even with a does that high, it did very little to elevate my Vitamin D levels. I later found that Vitamin D gets converted to its active form – also known as Calcitriol. Comparing with the thyroid mechanism we looked at earlier, this form of Vitamin D is what gets used by the cells. The Vitamin D receptors on the individual cells in the body actually recognize Calcitriol and not the Vitamin D that you ingest as food or supplements. The conversion of Vitamin D to Calcitriol happens in liver and kidneys. In my case, my Calcitriol values were much higher than the normal values and the Vitamin D values were lower than the reference ranges. What that indicated was that the issue was not with the Vitamin D consumption but in fact with how the Vitamin D was being utilized by my body. My cells were just not able to absorb the Vitamin D. This was the reason why even such a high dose of Vitamin D did not have much impact on my Vitamin D levels.

This was specifically my case, however, problems with Vitamin D cycles can be multi-faceted. There are multiple reasons why Vitamin D deficiency exists –

- You might not be getting enough of Vitamin D either through food, sunlight or supplements
- Your body might not be effectively converting Vitamin D to Calcitriol
- Your cells might not be able to absorb the Calcitriol due to multiple factors thus still giving out Vitamin D deficiency symptoms even when your Vitamin D intake is adequate.

When your Vitamin D intake is sufficient and the values are still showing up as deficient, it is important to have a discussion with the doctor and try to address the root cause.

One of the published hypothesis discusses the issue with Vitamin D toxicity in absence of Vitamin A or Vitamin K. In other words, it is believed and yet to be proved that Vitamin D supplementation by itself can actually cause Vitamin D toxicity since Vitamin D needs Vitamin A & K for metabolizing. Very recently there have been studies that are looking to either prove or disprove this hypothesis. One of the first studies out there published in October 2014 has found this to be an issue and has opened up the discussion for further studies around this. In any case, large doses of Vitamin D are something that you would want to be careful of especially when not accompanied by other fat soluble Vitamins such as A & K.

It is a very well-known fact that Vitamin D is produced naturally by the body when exposed to sunlight. However, when dealing with sun exposure, a lot of us are however also threatened by more complicated conditions such as skin cancer. In 2004, the American Journal of Clinical Nutrition, weighed in on this and found that a sensible sun exposure would be to get 5-10 minutes of exposure of arms and legs or hands, arms and face at least 2-3 times each week. This definitely does not sound a lot does it?

Now it is also important to note that Vitamin D is a fat soluble Vitamin. Which means that a significant amount of dietary fat is required for your body to absorb and utilize Vitamin D effectively. Furthermore, the CASPIAN III study done in Iran has demonstrated that a magnesium deficiency also causes Vitamin D deficiency. Hence, magnesium rich foods or supplementation also seems to be a key for avoiding Vitamin D deficiency.

Considering all these, a comprehensive diet, lifestyle and supplementation approach needs to be derived for addressing Vitamin D deficiency. First of all, you need to ensure that you are not on the low-fat bandwagon. Secondly, that there is enough magnesium-rich diet. Lastly, ensure that you have enough Vitamin D – ideally from sunlight but if not, from a good supplement that also provides Vitamin A & K.

Research Bits

Several studies have linked Vitamin D deficiency with auto-immunity. For instance, a Dec 2014 article from Australia titled "**Vitamin D and Immunity**" discusses this. Also, another article from Aug 2010 titled "**Vitamin D: modulator of the immune system**" reviews susceptibility of Vitamin D deficiency to chronic infections and auto-immunity.

The role of Vitamin K in avoiding Vitamin D toxicity is postulated in article titled "**Vitamin D toxicity redefined: vitamin K and the molecular mechanism**". Several other studies listed in references section discuss the relationship between Vitamin D with magnesium deficiency and stress responses.

All the studies can be found on pubmed.

Lab Tests

Most of the major labs in the US provide a blood test to check for Vitamin D levels. The tests can be ordered with a general physician or an endocrinologist.

Parasite Infections

Parasite infections are another big factor that can lead to a compromised intestinal barrier. Parasite infections can be caused due to hygiene factors or can be food or water borne.

Lab Tests

Most of the major labs in the US provide a blood test and a stool test to test for parasite infections. The tests can be ordered with a general physician or gastrointestinologist.

The treatment would differ based on the type of parasites identified. However, antibiotics should be avoided as much possible when curing such infections. Antibiotics are usually not targeted towards specific strains and hence can cause a significant degradation even in "good bacteria" population in the small intestine. If you recall our discussion earlier, the intestinal bacteria also play a role in conversion of the thyroid hormones and hence a healthy composition of the intestinal bacteria is essential to thyroid health. Antibiotics usually wipe out all the bacteria so the recovery for the thyroid protocol simply takes much longer time after antibiotic usage.

The partnership with the doctor

Once we understand the underlying causes, appropriate diet and lifestyle practices can be taken up to resolve the condition. As the body heals itself, there is an apparent need to adjust the dosage of the thyroid hormone to reflect the body's renewed ability to provide the hormone by itself. The typical thyroid dosage is usually just a single synthetic hormone replacement tablet. Hence, the modifications are usually not very complex and can be easily tracked.

When a change in the dosage of the thyroid hormone occurs, it takes the body 6-8 weeks for the complete impact on all the body functions to take place. Some patients see an immediate effect in mood, energy, hair quality and several other factors. However, it still does take 6-8 weeks for the effects to be seen throughout the body.

As you embark on these changes, it is recommended that you work with your endocrinologists to formulate an appropriate plan for tracking and adjusting the dosage. A comprehensive lab test of all the tests detailed below should be run every 6-8 weeks to track the changes and make appropriate changes in the hormone replacement dosage. At every step in this process, it is required to re-evaluate the dosage for synthetic thyroxin hormone been taken.

However, at no point should you stop taking the thyroid medication completely without a doctor intervention after reviewing the lab test results. The thyroid hormone is one of the important hormones for metabolism and unless the body's ability to generate its own thyroid hormones is completely restored, the synthetic hormones dosage must continue. A significant number of metabolic functions depend on the thyroid hormone making it a critical hormone for survival.

Below are some of the tests that you should be running on a regular basis once you start the process for healing your thyroid condition.

TSH	Thyroid Simulating Hormone. This is a primary marker that is usually used to determine the thyroid disorder.
Free T3	This marker looks at the amount of bio-available thyroid hormone T3 present in the blood that can be used by the cells
Free T4	This marker looks at the amount of bio-available thyroid hormone T4 present in the blood that can be used by the cells
TpoAB	Amount of Thyroid Peroxidase Antibodies in the blood.
TgAb	Amount of Thyroglobulin Antibodies in the blood.
Vitamin D	Vitamin D levels in the blood
HA1c	Also known as Glycated Hemoglobin, this measures the amount of blood sugar averaged out over approximately 3 months.

The human body typically has very small tolerances with these hormones, anti-bodies & vitamins. The lab values usually have very broad reference ranges. Hence, in order to ensure a right balance of these hormones while still working in boundaries of what modern medical tools can provide us, it is important to look at all these values in conjunction with each other and ensure that ALL the values fall in the right ranges.

Specific considerations however, need to be given to some of the values for which recent research suggests that the reference ranges might be out of the range the body is typically used to.

One such specific case will be for TSH values. The TSH reference ranges have changed significantly in last three decades. A few decades ago, the upper reference ranges were at 10 mIU/L. Over last several years, as more research keeps pouring in, these ranges have been adjusted to 4.5 mIU/L. However, even today, more research is being done to understand if these ranges need to be trimmed down further or least should be looked at along with other parameters including cardiovascular, metabolic or bone risk factors.

A recent article in Journal of Clinical Endocrinology and Metabolism takes a look at studies done in past decade to understand how the TSH reference values should be changed. One of the most striking aspects of the article was this revelation of how much disagreement is present amongst the medical research community itself around the appropriate values of TSH. The problem here in my opinion is that we are trying to look at a one size fits all approach which clearly isn't the most appropriate here. The article points to studies where higher normal values of TSH are linked to metabolic risk factors, coronary heart disease events and mortality. On the contrary, it also looks at very low level of TSH (rather below the reference range) to find correlations with a negative impact on cardiovascular health.

Understanding that there is still a limited body of knowledge around these values and even some conflicting evidences with that, I definitely expect the acceptable TSH ranges to keep getting revised over next several years as we get renewed understanding. At the same time, functional medicine practices seems to grasp the fact that the human body has a much stricter range than the currently acceptable vast range from 0.4 mUI/L to 4.5 mUI/L. However, I do not completely understand the basis behind those values and haven't seen much research supporting that. These however are still between the acceptable ranges of conventional medicine practice and hence possibly a much safer and reliable alternative to work with. Hence, a functional medicine doctor can very well help better interpret the values.

Considering the findings from the TSH reference range research paper as well as the learning from the functional medicine, if the TSH values on the lab tests start crossing the 2.5 mUI/L into the upper higher ranges, it is good to work with the doctor to understand if you are being more prone to any of the other disorders due to these values. The thyroid hormone replacement dosage can be adjusted to get this value in the appropriate range depending on the values seen with other tests such as Free T3 & Free T4.

It's probably best to partner with a functional medicine practitioner along with the regular endocrinologist.

▎Research Bits

The Journal of Clinical Endocrinology and Metabolism published an article titled "**The Normal TSH Reference Range: What has Changed in the last decade**". The article discusses studies around the TSH reference range and can be found in September 2013 issue of the journal.

When working on a corrective diet and lifestyle action for thyroid, multiple changes can be noted in the blood work that is done on regular basis. In order to mark good progress, it is highly recommended that a baseline of all these values be collected before making any changes. The regular blood work after each 6-8 weeks can then be compared with the baseline to get an idea of the progress being made. Keeping an eye on the progress is important in a lot of cases since it helps to continue working towards healing.

Some of the trends that can be observed are –

1) TPO & Tg Antibodies values decreasing: When we started making the diet and lifestyle changes which we will explore later in the book, the antibody numbers were significantly high. The TPO Antibodies were at 276 and the Tg antibodies were over 300. Within 6 months of following the protocol, the TPO antibodies were down to 7 & the Tg antibodies were down at 10. At this time, my TPO Antibodies are completely within the normal range and Tg antibodies are down to 7, still trending down. Do note however, that it took me almost 2 years to get to this state.

2) Decrease in TSH values: As the antibodies values start to decrease, a significant decrease in the TSH values is seen. The reason being that the thyroid hormones are still being compensated with synthetic hormone while the body is now able to prepare its own thyroid hormones. However, the body's own ability along with the unchanged external synthetic hormone dosage increases the Free T3 & T4 values in the bloodstream, hence, driving down the TSH values. In cases such as these, it is imperative to keep adjusting the thyroid hormone dosage to ensure that the TSH values are still kept in valid range. Some of the points mentioned above regarding the TSH values should be considered when making such a dosage change. As the TSH values decrease, do discuss with your doctor the possibility of reducing the synthetic thyroid hormone dosage with minimum variance possible so that the body is able to adapt without a shock. Thyroid is a critical hormone for metabolism and hence the changes should be gradual for the body to adjust.

Do expect this process to continue for a few years. Note that in most cases, the immune attacks on your thyroid started way before you realized that you had this condition. The thyroid gland has been inflamed for several years and hence, the healing process will be long as well.

Re-designing the Food Plate

"Let food by thy medicine and medicine be thy food"

- Hippocrates (460-377 B.C.)

What Hippocrates preached several thousand years ago was similar to the fundamentals of Ayurveda. When medicine progressed as science on the principles of reductionism, we lost some of the ancient wisdom that kept us free of the modern diseases seen today. While we made significant progress eradicating some of the deadliest of the diseases, we are quickly succumbing to the diseases of the modern civilization.

The subsequent chapters explores the concepts of nourishing the body with good food. We look at what a nourishing plate looks like, what are the foods to avoid and some tips on what the shopping cart should look like when you go shopping for food.

It is important to understand that all these changes can very rarely be implemented at once. It will usually take a few months or even years to completely implement some of the changes discussed here. The over reliance on packaged & processed foods makes this even more challenging. However, the key is to keep making incremental changes and easing into the changed lifestyle every time a change is made.

The body presents layers of security barriers for foreign elements before they can reach inside to cause any damage. The skin is by far the most visible of these barriers and does a fantastic job of keeping most of the pathogens out of reach. The entire pathway through which the food travels presents another such barrier for whatever is ingested. If you look closely, the mouth, esophagus, stomach, small and large intestine provide a passage for the externally ingested food to travel through the body while carefully extracting the required nutrients at each step. Anything that is deemed dangerous for the body is immediately eliminated through this pathway by means of stools. Ever wondered why eating contaminated food results the diarrhea? That's the body's way of protecting itself. The intestine thus acts as a second major barrier for the body. Some of the other such barriers are the lungs & the brain as well. The lungs keep pollutants from air from entering the parts of the body whereas the barrier of the brain barrier protects the brain even when the toxins are able to enter the body through breaking these other barriers.

In some of the previous chapters, we already explored how the compromising of the intestinal lining is one of the biggest contributors to auto-immunity. No surprises that healing this lining is one of the first and key steps in moving towards a better health with auto-immunity. In the previous chapter we looked at how to identify some of the foods that can be causing an impact to the gut lining. It's is important to understand that apart from those foods, any foods or substances that are unidentifiable by the body are very likely to cause inflammation in the gut. Also, the overall inflammation in the body causes the intestinal lining to break and it is hence very important to control the inflammation as well.

Healing the intestinal lining is a two-step process. In the first step, it is important to completely remove the foods that would cause stress on the digestion process. Secondly, also introduce foods and lifestyle changes that heal this lining. Lifestyle changes also need to be introduced to reduce the overall stress since stress is also a major contributor to a compromised gut.

The effects of diet for resolving the intestinal permeability and minimizing the immune attack on the thyroid are multiplied when combined with the right lifestyle changes. Our habits around Sleep, Exercise & movement, stress management also have a significant impact on the foods that we crave for and eat. Hence, taking care of these factors also provides us with the ability to much easily stick to the diet changes. Chapters after the dietary changes are focused on Lifestyle changes. These, together with the diet changes would provide great results for the thyroid function.

Gluten

Gluten seems to be emerging as by far one of the most pervasive foods today that impacts the gut. Dr. William Davis discusses this in his book "The Wheat Belly". He attributes this in part to the rampant hybridization of the grain for bigger yields that has led to it becoming almost a completely new strain of grain that the body no longer recognizes.

The average consumption of wheat and related grains has steadily increased in last several decades. A breakfast today very commonly starts with a slice of bread or a donut, followed by a sandwich for lunch & pasta or bread again for dinner. These are just the macro constituents on the food plate. Food manufacturers & restaurants have introduced gluten as a binding agent or thickening agent in variety of different foods which you would generally not even think of being related to gluten or grains – for instance, various sauces, soups, chocolates, flavored milk powders, spices such as asafetida and many more. As a result, gluten forms over almost 40% of our calorie intake today. This is a substantial increase in just last 50 years after the packaged food industry took over.

The combination of the hybridization process and a sudden increase in consumption has almost taken the body by surprise – not giving it enough time to evolve itself to adapt to the changing circumstances. Moreover, changing agricultural practices are not helping either. Just 50 years ago, there was not a thing such as organic farming. Everything that was being farmed was of course without pesticides. World War II and the Cold War after that saw the advent of pesticides and pesticides based farming. It took several decades after that before farming practices even tried to go back to the way it was before.

Apart from what Dr. William Davis discusses in his book about gluten intolerance, glyphosate – an active component of herbicide Round-up. Although, glyphosate has been declared safe for humans by Monsanto (who incidentally has their entire business model based off glyphosate), there are scattered studies in the scientific community that explores glyphosate and its impact on the body. These studies have seen impact on intestinal cells and cardiovascular functions. The 2005 study in Canada shows a disruption in barrier properties of the intestinal cells and hence has a potential for direct impact on intestinal permeability.

Glyphosate is usually used along with the GMO crops. However, some recent agricultural practices suggest that glyphosate is now being used with wheat fields, mostly as weed killer just before the sowing, but also in some cases just before the harvest. Some theories say that this leads to a very high glyphosate content in the wheat that is produced.

Given all these factors, gluten today is one of the major offenders of the leaky gut. For me, after almost a decade of disease progression, getting rid of gluten showed me results in just more than a month. Eliminating gluten helped me get my thyroid anti-bodies values down to almost normal.

▌ Research Bits

A 2005 study done in Canada explores impact of Glyphosate on intestinal lining. This study is titled "**Oral bioavailability of glyphosate: studies using two intestinal**

61

cell lines". Another Sep 2014 article review all the literature that associates glyphosate with cardiovascular risks and demands further studies on the subject. This article is titled **"Glyphosate-Based Herbicides Potently Affect Cardiovascular System in Mammals: Review of the Literature"**. Both these can be found on pubmed.

The pervasiveness of gluten in our diet makes gluten free living a tough challenge. When we decided to go gluten free after looking at all the data and evidences, it took us almost 3 months to prepare ourselves and work our way towards a complete elimination from our diets. The stocked shelves in the supermarket don't help either. Gluten has been shown to have addictive qualities which make it harder to quit.

While you work your way towards a gluten free world, there are several important changes that need to be considered.

- What are all the places in your existing diet where wheat or gluten is pervasive?
- What do you replace gluten with?
- What are some of the commonly consumed packaged foods?

The first question is probably easily answered by looking at your current typical food plate. Some of the most common offenders are obvious – bread, pasta, cakes, pastries, pizza. Eliminating these would probably take care of over 95% of your gluten intake. However, the remaining 5% sometimes needs you to assume a role of an investigative journalist. Start reading the ingredient labels on everything. Some of the common places on the ingredient labels that directly translate to gluten are –

- All-purpose Flour
- Wheat
- Barley
- Rye
- Spelt
- Wheat Protein / Hydrolyzed Wheat Protein
- Wheat Starch
- Wheat Flour
- Bread Flour
- Bleached Flour
- Malt
- Bulgur

Apart from some of these direct ingredients, there are several ingredients that can be derived from gluten. Food laws permit the manufacturers to not disclose the ingredients in Natural & Artificial Flavorings since these are typically the "trade secrets". In a lot of cases, such flavorings can be derived from wheat or barley making it further difficult to experience benefits of going completely gluten free. A safer way to avoid gluten is to pick up processed foods that are explicitly marked gluten free.

The "Gluten-Free" labeling refers to any food product that contains less than 20 parts per million of gluten. The FDA recently standardized the definition of gluten free requiring the foods marked as "no gluten", "free of gluten" and "without gluten" to meet the definition of "gluten-free".

| Research Bits

The FDA defines gluten free if the food does not contain wheat, rye, barley or any cross breeds of these grains. It also mandates that the foods should not contain more than 20 ppm of gluten. A quick search for gluten on the FDA website (www.fda.gov) provides good information about the labeling laws.

Not surprisingly, as more and more people get on the gluten-free bandwagon, the market is responding swiftly. Gluten free options are flooding the store shelves and restaurant menus. The gluten containing grains usually tend to make sticky dough. Thus making them best suitable for making breads and cakes and similar foods. The alternative ingredients used typically do not provide the sticky texture that is needed for most of such items. Hence, the "gluten-free" foods in restaurants or market shelves tend to be a mixture of more than one ingredients that substitute gluten.

Some of the common alternative ingredients are –

- Corn Starch
- White Rice Flour
- Brown Rice Flour
- Tapioca Flour
- Potato Starch
- Xanthum Guam
- Guar Gum

Although these ingredients do not contain gluten, they cause a similar gastrointestinal distress due to their highly processed nature and high glycemic loads. Since the key objective of removing gluten is to relieve the small intestine of constant attack, it is highly recommended that such processed foods be avoided as well.

Several websites and cook books advocating a gluten free lifestyle today provide easy recipes for common comfort foods using alternative ingredients such as almond flour & eggs as a binding agent. Such recipes usually have a lower shelf life and hence are not found on the super market stores. Getting in the kitchen and preparing the food the old fashioned heart and soul way is probably the most effective way of going gluten free.

Sugar

Sugar is another major contributor to the leaky gut. In fact, the devastating impact of sugar goes much beyond just the gut. For people familiar with Diabetes, sugar is definitely not a stranger. Several recent studies have found very high correlation between elevated blood glucose levels and thyroid disorders. Although science does understand the correlation here, the cause of mechanism of how blood glucose impacts the thyroid function is still being debated within the research circles. But a significant correlation was enough for a 2010 review study from Prince Charles Hospital, UK to suggest that all the diabetes patients be routinely checked for thyroid dysfunctions. This recommendation is sufficient to indicate a strong correlation and perhaps enough to stress on the importance of managing the blood glucose levels for thyroid disorders.

Looking back at my personal experience, this might also be the reason why I was suffering from polycystic ovarian syndrome (PCOS). The PCOS is known to be a combination of impaired blood glucose metabolism and thyroid imbalances.

This book does not focus a lot on blood glucose control. There is a vast collection of literature out there around Diabetes and blood sugar management which can be relied on for this purpose. However, given the importance of this parameter for intestinal and overall thyroid health, this chapter will discuss ways to avoid added sugars in the diet. Added sugars are by far the most important aspect of blood glucose management. There are several other strategies including lowering of carbohydrates in the diet – which in fact the American Diabetes Association now recommends.

However, that of course would be a discussion separate from this book. For most of the people who are not on external insulin medication, removal of added sugars can substantially help manage the blood glucose levels and assist with the healing of the thyroid condition.

Contrary to a popular belief that we need sugar for energy, we do get enough sugar from our usual carbohydrate intake to sustain throughout the day. In fact, since we completely eliminated sugar for over a year now, we are experiencing high and sustained energy throughout the day. Having seen what sugar can do to the otherwise healthy energy levels, I can now safely make a statement that any amount of added sugar beyond the usual carbohydrate intake should be seen as unnecessary or even harmful to the body.

Eliminating sugar however is much trickier – again due to the pervasive nature of sugar and also due to its addictive nature. One such study compares the addictive nature of sugar to that of cocaine describing it to be "even more rewarding and attractive" than cocaine. Sugar addiction works by increasing the dopamine activity in the brain. Dopamine the chemical in the brain responsible for feelings such as motivation, cognition and reward. Dopamine dysfunctions are also related to other brain diseases such as Parkinsons and Schizophrenia and studies are underway to determine if sugar or excess carbohydrates intake might have a direct linkage to such diseases.

| Research Bits

The International Journal of Clinical Practice published a review study in July 2010 titled "**Thyroid dysfunction in patients with diabetes: clinical implications and screening**

strategies". This review emphasizes the strong correlation between diabetes and thyroid. It also recommends a routine thyroid check-up for all the diabetes patients. A similar study performed in Czech Republic in 2005 recommended screening for thyroid for all the Type II Diabetes patients. This study was titled "**Thyroid gland diseases in adult patients with diabetes mellitus**"

The American Heart Association now advises against added sugar. A 2005 study titled "**Cardiovascular risk factors in children with Type 1 Diabetes and their relationship with the glycemic control**" clearly discusses the increased cardiovascular risk associated with high blood sugars.

University of Roma, Italy, published an article in March 2014 titled "**Sugar and Chromosome Stability**". This discusses a strong link between Sugar and Cancer.

University of Bordeaux, France published two studies in 2007 & 2008 that discusses the addictive nature of sugar. These studies compared sugar with cocaine and found sugar to be even more addictive than cocaine. The studies titled "**Intense Sweetness surpasses cocaine reward**" & "**Evidence for Sugar Addiction: behavioral and neurochemical effects of intermittent, excessive sugar intake**" can be found on Pubmed.

When it comes to sugar, the packaged food manufacturers are at no mercy. Sugar hides under a variety of different names such as –

- High fructose Corn Syrup
- Evaporated Cane Juice
- Beet Sugar
- Cane Sugar
- Cane Juice Crystals
- Corn Syrup

- Confectioner's Sugar
- Dextrose
- Fructose
- Fruit Juice Concentrate
- Glucose
- Glucose Solids
- Maltodextrin
- Molasses
- Refiner's Syrup
- Sucrose
- Brown Rice Sugar
- Raw Sugar.

The list continues lot more with new creative names added every day. To think about it, a confectioner's sugar or refiner's sugar is just that – Sugar. The process of preparing sugar from sugar cane involves juicing the sugarcane and evaporating it to form sugar crystals. No surprise that a healthy sounding name such as "Evaporated Sugarcane juice" is really the plain old sugar. When it comes to sugar, organic is not good either – Organic sugar is still sugar for the body – nothing better.

In addition to the creative naming, sugar is also added to foods that you would never expect to have sugar. For instance, one of the ingredients in the "healthy" brown bread is the high fructose corn syrup (HFCS). The HFCS is also an ingredient in a regular tomato ketchup & even in children's medication. Not just that, just an 8 oz glass of the healthy looking juice has at least 22 grams of sugar or 5 /12 teaspoons of sugar. The American Heart Association recommends not having more than 6 teaspoons of sugar each day for women. A glass of the so called healthy fruit juice takes you right through your recommended intake of sugar. Thoroughly reading and understanding ingredient labels is probably the best defense against sugar.

Getting rid of sugar, gets us out of almost 90% of the packaged foods available. This also helps us move majority of our food intake towards fresh vegetables and meat – which in turn helps turn away from the sugar addiction. When going sugar free however, it is also important to understand that the alternatives if at all should be carefully picked. The low calorie sweetener alternatives are used for several years in the mainstream and have gained a controversial reputation. A recent study for instance, evaluated Aspartame and found it to be having a neurobehavioral impact. Participants consuming aspartame were seen to be having irritable moods, depression & worsened spatial orientation. This probably indicates that there is some level of influence aspartame has on the brain. However, this is contradicted by another recent study that examines multiple studies since 1990 to 2012 and concludes that aspartame is safe. Hence, when it comes to sugar alternatives, it is probably safe to stick to natural sugars such as fruits or honey or dates. Even with these, the guidance should be minimum possible consumption of such natural sweeteners. It should be of significant note that most of the drinks labeled as "Diet" use some form of artificial sweeteners and hence should be avoided as much as possible.

Research Bits

The Food and Chemical Toxicology published an Italian review in October 2013. The study titled **"Aspartame, low-calorie sweeteners and disease:**

regulatory safety and epidemiological issues" reviews all the studies concerning Aspartame from 1990 to 2012 and found no significant risk of cancers and pregnancy related disorders. The study can be found on Pubmed.

Another study by University of North Dakota published in April 2014 finds impact of aspartame on neurobehavioral health. The study titled **"Neurobehavioral Effects of Aspartame Consumption"** can be found on Pubmed.

Soy

Soy is usually considered a health food. Tofu, Soy Milk have recently been highly popular in health circles. However, for those with thyroid disorders, Soy seems to have several negative effects. Studies show that soy interferes with the thyroid absorption. This has specifically seen to be the case with individuals that are already taking doses of levothyroxine. A 2012 study done in the Pediatric department of University of California in San Diego has found the Soy to be having detrimental effect on thyroid in pediatrics. The thyroid function was seen to improve significantly in the infants when the soy formula was either stopped or changed to cow milk. Another rat study published in July 2014 also found negative impact of Soy on normal thyroid function.

When we look at the traditional eastern cultures where soy consumption was much more common than anywhere else, we see that the way soy was consumed was much different than today. Soy used to be usually consumed after fermentation and were consumed in far lesser quantities than what we have today. This of course presents a different set of challenges for our body since it is not used to such high consumption especially without fermentation. Fermentation of the Soy would've usually made it much more easily digestable by our body, thus reduce the negative effects that Soy would've otherwise had. Soy today is widely used not just as Tofu or Soy Milk, but also used as an emulsifier in variety of packaged foods. Thus, our consumption of Soy today is much higher and in much processed form that what our bodies are suited for.

Therefore, at least for people with hypothyroidism, Soy is best avoided in any of the forms. Packaged foods containing Soy products such as Soy lecithin should be avoided as well.

Research Bits

Multiple studies have explored the impact of Soy on the thyroid function. Two of the studies noted here can be found on pubmed. These are titled – **"Soy isoflavones interfere with thyroid hormone homeostasis in orchidectomized middle-aged rats"** and **"Unawareness of the effects of soy intake on the management of congenital hypothyroidism"**

Reduce Toxicity from Food

Toxicity from food is often a topic of a hearty debate. Conventional agriculture harnesses the power of chemistry to improve the yields year over year and help the noble cause of world hunger. While several advocates of the world hunger also say that we already grow much more than is required to feed the world, we however, need to fix the food supply chain. Although solving world hunger is quite out of context of this book, the use of chemicals in forms of pesticides, fungicides and herbicides is definitely a concern when it comes to overall intestinal health.

Chemicals used to grow the food today, are by far some of the dangerous chemical substances for human health. In one of his talks, Michael Pollan, an American author and journalists, describes pesticides used in Idaho for potato crops. He mentions that the pesticides are so dangerous that the farmers do not enter their own fields for almost a week after spraying it.

There are several studies discussing the toxic effects of such pesticides on the body. One such study conducted in India discusses the impact of common pesticides on the metabolism and specifically on the thyroid hormone receptors on cells. In this study pesticides were seen to have affinity towards the thyroid hormone receptors thus causing hypothyroidism. These thyroid disrupting pesticides can also disrupt the overall metabolic regulation thus causing weight gain, lethargy and other similar issues. Another article published by the University of California, LA discusses the thyroid hormone suppression behavior due to pesticides and several other components.

Recent research in the genetics has shown us that the genes that we think of as "inherited" and "set in stone" are in fact much more fluid and change according to our diet and lifestyle changes. This interesting field of study is called epigenetics. Combining the epigenetics with nutrition has also led to an emergence of Nutrigenomics. Nutrigenomics explores the effects of nutrients on genomes and the interaction between diet and disease and genetic links in between. A 2004 abstract on Pubmed titled "Nutrigenomics and Nutrigenetics" discusses a possibility of using nutrition towards epigenetics and disease remediation. Although this is a very new and emerging field with very less evidence of its success, the exploration of this possibility tells me that we do not yet completely understand how food impacts the body. Food is definitely much more than calories. It has been seen as signals of information to the genes that then direct the mechanisms in body to do certain activities and demonstrate certain behaviors.

Genetically modified or GMO foods are foods that are genetically modified in the laboratory. It is said that GMO holds a promise of potentially solving world hunger. In the light of emerging sciences such as Nutrigenomics, where we acknowledge that we do not completely understand how food and its processing impacts our body, I see GMOs as a substantial risk putting one more ball in the air in the already complex world of nutrition and disease management. If GMOs help solve the world hunger or not remains to be seen. However, for whatever it is worth, I do consider GMOs out of equation when trying to optimize diet for a healthy gut & thyroid functioning simply because of all the unknowns around it.

Here in the US, the USDA defines a standard for "Organic". Thankfully the standard does not include either pesticides or GMO foods. Hence, when it comes to reducing the toxicity of food, Organic food becomes a de-facto choice.

The debate between organic and non-organic is not really of a nutritional value. It is about getting least harmful impact from the foods.

▎Research Bits

The **USDA National Organic Program** defines the organic standards for not just the crops but also for animals and multi-ingredient foods.

Organic crops prohibit use of pesticides or GMO. Organic livestock ensures a 100% organic feed for the animals without the use of antibiotics or hormones. Multi-ingredient foods (packaged foods) that are labels organic are required to have at least a 95% or more certified organic content.

A study published by University of Allahabad, India in Feb 2014 discusses how pesticides can cause metabolic disruptions and hypothyroidism even in low doses. The study is titled "**Pesticides in mixture disrupt metabolic regulation**" and can be searched on Pubmed.

A 2010 article by UCLA discusses how pesticides (and several other environmental factors) cause suppression in thyroid hormones. The article titled "**Environment Exposures and Autoimmune Thyroid Disease**" can be found on Pubmed.

Apart from some of these obvious toxicity concerns from GMO & pesticides, foods today need much more scrutiny, thanks for the growing processing on the foods.

For instance, MSG or Monosodium Glutamate is a very common flavor enhancing additive to a lot of processed & restaurant foods these days. This additive has been recognized for its neurotoxic effects. However, it still slips into the processed foods under variety of different names since it is a low cost flavor enhancer – probably even an addictive. Similar to MSG, processed foods have several other added chemicals today that the body is unable to identify and process. Consumption of such foods, leads to a series of cascading effects in the body, starting as fundamental as gut imbalances to something really complex as brain toxicity.

The Monosodium Glutamate (MSG) is a very common flavor enhancer being used in packaged and canned foods since last several decades. Some people are sensitive or even allergic to MSG. However, most of the population does not have any direct symptoms when consuming MSG. However, multiple studies allude to neurological (brain related) toxicity

& even toxicity to the fetus of the brain in pregnant women due to MSG. Although the Food and Drug Administration (FDA) does not categorize MSG as a banned or even a potentially harmful substance, studies & reviews do seem to indicate that the verdict for MSG is not out yet. While some studies have seen correlation in neurological toxicity, it is yet to be seen on what other organs it impacts. Given the potentially toxic nature, foods containing MSG should definitely be removed off the list when healing the body. In packaged foods today, MSG is reported on the ingredients lists with multiple names –

- Glutamic Acid
- Yeast Extract
- Autolyzed Yeast
- Hydrolyzed Vegetable Protein
- Hydrolyzed Animal Protein

According to one of the articles by Vanderbuilt University, anything Ultra-Pasteurized or anything enzyme-modified can also contain MSG due to the processing involved.

Defenders of MSG also argue with the fact that MSG is an integral part of certain vegetables such as tomato. But what they fail to mention is that the quantity of MSG in a tomato is a significantly lower than what you find in most processed foods. While the natural vegetables might have this compound in insignificant quantities, I have seen certain Chinese restaurants use it by spoonfuls.

> ▍Research Bits
>
> A study conducted in Saudi Arabia in March 2014 looks at the effects of MSG on certain cognitive functions. The study titled **"Cognitive and**

biochemical effects of monosodium glutamate and aspartame, administered individually and in combination in male albino mice" can be found on Pubmed.

Another 1994 study done in China found neurotoxic effects in mice babies in the womb due to MSG consumed by the mother. This study is titled "**Transplacental neurotoxic effects of monosodium glutamate on structures and functions of specific brain areas of filial mice**"

Another important factor to look at when reducing the toxicity from the foods is the artificial food colors and flavors. Food colors and flavors are those that are added to the food items most often to simulate the presence of fresh fruits and vegetables. These are usually used in lieu of the actual fruits or vegetables in order to lower the cost of the food items. Food colors today are fairly pervasive with the packaged foods. Most of the food colors have a petro-chemicals based and are known have detrimental effects on brain, liver and kidneys. As for the direct impact on thyroid, there are is only a single study on pubmed that explores the effects of artificial food coloring and flavoring on thyroid and does find detrimental effects. However, this study was done back in 1991. Given that it has been over 23 years since the study was published, there might be significant changes to how the food coloring and flavoring is now manufactured. Hence, we do not know as of now how much relevant that study is. However, we have seen that the thyroid gland does not work in isolation. It requires a healthy functioning of intestines and liver in order to convert the T4 hormones to T3 and aid in the overall thyroid cycle.

Some recent studies do find that the food colors and flavors do have a detrimental effect on the liver.

The detrimental impact of food dyes and flavoring is very commonly known in the European Union to an extent that the food dyes are banned for the most part throughout the European countries. However, these still remain in the mainstream market here in the United States. The Center for Science in Public Interest (http://www.cspinet.org/fooddyes/) has filed multiple petitions with the food manufacturers to remove these colorings from the food items – especially those targeted to smaller children.

Some of the common food dyes found on the packaged foods are –

- Red 40
- Yellow 5
- Yellow 6
- Red 3
- Orange B
- Green 3
- Citrus Red 2
- Blue 1
- Blue 2

Apart from the studies found on Pubmed, the Center for Science in Public Interest (CSPI) has published a PDF called "Rainbow of Risks" that summarizes the latest research around the toxicity of these artificial coloring. In this paper, you can see that the Red 3 color is shown to cause Thyroid Cancers in some rat studies. Other colors such as Yellow 5 and Yellow 6 are shown to contain carcinogenic contaminants. Yellow 5 is also shown to cause hyperactivity disorders in children.

Given the impact of these color and flavors, for optimal thyroid functioning, it is best to avoid these wherever possible.

▌Research Bits

The Center for Science in Public Interest has published an article called "**Food Dyes:Rainbow of Risks**". This can be found by a simple Internet Search.
Another 2013 study from Egypt finds significant impact on blood and liver from the food colorings. This study titled "**Toxic effects of some synthetic food colorants and/or flavor additives on male rats**" can be found on pubmed.

Gut Healing Foods

Once the foods that promote gut inflammation are removed, the next step towards healing the gut is to actually introduce foods and changes that would heal it. Healing of the gut is an important part of fighting back the auto-immunity. As you would visualize intestinal permeability, while the leakiness exists, the un-digested foods will keep slipping in the blood stream. Hence, it is imperative to plug the holes and ensure a healthy functioning gut in order to counter auto-immune conditions.

As a gut healing food, my introduction to the bone broth was really from the alternate medicine after I read Dr. Allison Siebecker's article in the 2005 (Feb/Mar) of the Townsend Letter. As I started doing more food anthropological research starting from this article, I realized that bone broth at one point in history was a very commonly used food. Dr. Weston A. Price talks about this in his book "Nutrition and Physical Degeneration" about the benefits of bone broth. Gelatin and even bone broth to some extent, was studied in the medical community till almost 1950s. After that period however, there seems to be a significant decrease in the any scientific investments in studying this food. Connecting the dots with some of the recent studies along with the older ones, bone broth however does seem a very logical food to be used in healing intestinal problems. For instance, a 1934 study conducted by Kings College Hospital, London looks at bone broth to find that its protein is mainly constituted of gelatin. Another recent study done in 2013 by Kyoto University, Japan discusses how gelatin can be used for healing Anastomotic leakage after intestinal surgery. Anastomotic leakage is basically a complication occurring from the intestinal surgeries where the intestines basically "leak" due to the post effects of surgery. Joining the dots here, which might seem a bit far-fetched, but bone broth does seem to offer a natural food solution for intestinal leakiness. Combining this with anthropological studies of traditional diets where bone broth was heavily used, it definitely seems a logical conclusion.

The bone broth is basically a broth or soup made by simmering the animal bones in water for long time (typically over 12-48 hours). Such broth, is usually rich in gelatin, which has been found to be promising to heal the leakiness of intestines after intestinal surgery etc. The broth can be easily made at home with several recipes available online. Getting it in store is a bit tricky though. Some of the store brands usually are using MSG (monosodium glutamate) for the flavorings or some other chemicals and additives for extending the shelf life. This counters the benefits offered by this food. Buying bone broth, either in store or online should definitely be whetted out to ensure that it does not contain some of these chemicals or additives that might in fact end up irritating the gut lining rather than helping it heal. However, bone broth prepared from organic animal sources and free of any chemicals such as MSG is definitely a great food for healing.

This has very quickly become a common food in our kitchen. At multiple times, I have used this myself for healing after strenuous workouts or to prevent an onset of cold or flu right after the first symptoms.

> ▌Research Bits
>
> The 1934 study exploring nutrient value in bone broth is titled "**Bone and Vegetable Broth**" and can be found on Pubmed.

The University of Kyoto, Japan published a study in October 2013 that looked at how gelatin can be useful in healing the intestine. This study titled **"Enhanced intestinal anastomotic healing with gelatin hydrogel incorporating basic fibroblast growth factor**" can be searched on Pubmed.

Dr. Allison Siebecker's article in Townsend Letter in the Feb-March 2005 edition titled "**Traditional Bone Broth in Modern Health and Disease**" provides great information on the nutritional content of this food and its impact on diseases and normal body functions.

Turmeric is another such food that is known to have a similar gut healing effect. Turmeric is a very well-known herb Indian medicine & extremely common spice in Indian food. In recent years, the active ingredient of turmeric – Curcumin – has been a subject of a lot of research, after it was discovered to be helping with cancer treatments. It is perhaps these cancer treatments that have led to finding some of the most interesting effects in non-cancer patients.

One of the treatments of cancer is chemotherapy. As you might already be aware, Chemotherapy usually has very intense effects on the body and hence has significantly impacted its effectiveness. One of the big side-effects of chemotherapy is intestinal dysfunction. Leaky gut or a compromised intestinal lining is one of the biggest impact on the intestine. In some of the mouse studies, curcumin was seen to improve the condition of the small intestine and almost heal the intestinal lining or at the least prevent it from breaking down completely. Other similar studies explore the use of curcumin for intestinal permeability induced due to drugs used for managing auto-immune conditions.

Furthermore, curcumin is also known to be a very good anti-inflammatory. Continuous inflammation has been shown to increase intestinal permeability. Hence, curcumin also works to reduce the stress on the intestinal lining by reducing inflammation.

> ▎ Research Bits
>
> Two recent studies done in China explore the benefits of curcumin for intestinal permeability induced due to drugs used for chemotherapy. These studies can be found on Pubmed. The titles for these are "**Protective effect of Curcumin on chemotherapy-induced intestinal dysfunction**" and "**Protective effect of curcumin against methotrexate-induced small intestinal damage in rats**"

It is said that the human body comprises of more bacteria and other micro-organisms than the human cells. There are several billion more bacteria in the body when compared with the human cells. Recently an article on NY Times written by Michael Pollan really hit this point hard with a set of very compelling evidences. As a part of medical research, we are just now starting to understand the important of gut microbes and its impact on the overall body. For instance, a part of thyroid hormone conversion from T4 to T3 also occurs in the gut in presence of specific enzymes and the gut microbes. These gut microbes or the gut flora also provide a good healing grounds for the intestinal permeability. Essentially, the gut cannot be healed without considering the effects of the gut flora. The intestinal flora represents a wide variety of bacteria. Imagine more than thousands of bacterial species living symbiotically within the very walls of your gut. The term probiotics usually refers to these bacteria. The probiotic supplements usually contain billions of bacteria that belong very few number of strains. This essentially starts compromising the variety of the bacteria hindering some of the functions that the other strains are taking care of.

Mainstream medicine is now starting to understand the importance of a rich healthy intestinal flora. A recent study done in China discusses how specific bacterial strains can be useful in healing the leaky gut. The studies also observed that a combination of multiple strains of bacteria is much more potent in healing than any single strain. Given that the probiotic supplements usually target only specific strains of bacteria, it is important to start looking at food or nutrition as the source of probiotics rather than probiotic supplements. Fermented foods such as Yogurt, Kefir, Sauerkraut, Pickles, Cheese, Buttermilk, Kombucha, Kvass etc. provide a natural way of introducing probiotics in the foods.

Again, when purchasing some of these foods in the store, it is important to ensure that they are not added with additives or ingredients to increase the shelf life. In most of the cases, such foods are very easily prepared at home with minimal effort.

Managing the variety of intestinal bacteria is not just limited to ingesting more of the probiotic foods. Another way of improving this bacterial ecosystem is by using what is called as "prebiotics". The prebiotics can be thought of as food for the bacteria within the intestines. The prebiotics generally promote the growth of such bacterial colonies thus helping a healthy intestine. The overall knowledge about the prebiotics in the medical science community is in very early stages as of now. There have been a few animal and human studies that seem to suggest that prebiotics can be helpful to counteract diseases such as diabetes, metabolic syndromes as well as cancer.

Nutritional science now recognizes Resistant Starches for their prebiotic capabilities. Resistant starches are the components in foods that would go undigested in the intestine. They are able to react with certain enzymes within the intestines to create fuel sources or foods for the bacteria living there. Some of the common foods that contain resistant starches are –

- Brown Rice
- Unripe Bananas
- Beans
- Legumes
- Potatoes

Do note however that of all the starches in these foods, only 5% are resistant starches. Over consumption of these foods still results in the remaining 95% starches getting converted to glucose and impacting the blood sugar.

❚ Research Bits

A recent study done in China, published in March 2014, discusses the role of probiotics in healing the intestinal barrier or the leaky gut. This study titled **"Are there any different effects of Bifidobacterium, Lactobacillus and Streptococcus on intestinal sensation, barrier function and intestinal immunity in PI-IBS mouse model?"** can be searched on Pubmed.

Another study from Italy, published in October 2013 reviews some of the work done earlier in counteracting diseases such as diabetes & cancer with prebiotics and acknowledges that the effect of the prebiotics might really be much broader than what the medical science previously thought. This study titled **"Prebiotics to fight diseases: reality or fiction?"** can be found on Pubmed.

Foods that Impact Thyroid Function

Some foods, based on their contents, can actually impact the thyroid function in a positive of negative way. In most cases, these are the foods that have certain elements that are used by the thyroid process itself – either by the gland or by some other organs that are responsible for converting the thyroid hormones. In other cases, the effect is not that direct but still quite significant.

Cruciferous Vegetables

If you have read about managing thyroid earlier, this is definitely something that you have come across. The term cruciferous refers to a class of vegetables such as cauliflower, broccoli, cabbage, bok choy, brussels sprouts and similar. Cruciferous vegetables are considered goitrogenic. In other words, they interfere with iodine uptake, thus negatively impacting the thyroid function. This usually causes a lower production of thyroid thus raising the TSH values. The cruciferous vegetables can be cooked to reduce the goitrogenic effect. So although you do not want to consume any of the cruciferous vegetables raw, these foods can certainly find place in the diet in the cooked form.

Other Foods

The process of producing the thyroid hormone and delivering it to the individual cells is a multi-step process. We covered that in one of the previous chapters. Each step depends on certain key bio-chemicals that in-turn depend on certain nutrients that we get from our food. An inefficiency at any of these steps due to nutrient scarcity in the body can mean inefficient delivery of thyroid hormones to the individual cells in the body. Thus triggering an elevated TSH release and symptoms of hypothyroidism.

Recent research has definitely taken a lot of inspiration from the ancient medicinal practices. Ashwagandha is a traditional Indian herb. Also known as Indian Ginseng or Winter Cherry, this herb has been used since centuries in ancient Indian medical practice of Ayurveda. The research has recently caught up to quantify the impact that this herb has on the thyroid. Studies from India have shown that Ashwagandha stimulates thyroid activity by enhancing serum T4 concentrations. Unlike the supplemental dose of levothyroxine, this herb is known to boost the body's own ability for producing the T4 hormone. Thus reducing the need for additional supplementation. The dosage tested in these studies was 2.5 mg per kg of bodyweight. For most of us, this translates to 150 mg to 250 mg per day. Most of the Ashwagandha capsules available in the market today are well within this range. However, there is one case study of a Dutch women who developed Thyroidtoxicosis when on supplementation containing Ashwagandha. This is just a single person case study, however, it is definitely recommended to introduce this herb in consideration with a naturopathic doctor or a practitioner who is qualified in administering herbs.

The thyroid gland itself, depends on Iodine & an amino acid called Tyrosine to produce the thyroid hormones. Perhaps the easiest way to bump up the Iodine intake is to use the Iodized salt. Alternatively, foods grown in and around the sea such as natural sea salt, sea weed etc are also very rich sources of Iodine. The other raw material for the thyroid hormones, Tyrosine is an amino acid. Tyrosine rich foods include poultry, dairy, nuts and seeds.

At various different stages in the body, the thyroid hormone T4, gets converted into its more readily bio-available form – T3. One such conversion happens in the liver. The conversion process of T4 to T3 in the liver relies on certain enzymes that require Selenium. Hence, the deficiency of Selenium in the food can also adversely impact the thyroid processes. Selenium is available in trace amounts in lot of different foods. But in order to really elevate the Selenium levels in the body, you would want to resort to foods high in Selenium such as Brazil Nuts or salt water fish such as Tuna, Halibut, Sardines or Shrimps. A very recent September 2014 study has explored Selenium as a treatment option for thyroid Hashimoto's and found it to be fairly promising.

Research Bits

Multiple studies out of India have explored the use of Ashwagandha for thyroid. Two such studies that I looked into are titled "**Withania somnifera and Bauhinia purpurea in the regulation of circulating thyroid hormone concentrations in female mice**" and "**Changes in thyroid hormone concentrations after administration of ashwagandha root extract to adult male mice**".
Another study published in September 2014 explores the use of Selenium for treating Hashimoto's. This study is titled "**The importance of Selenium in Hashimoto's disease**". All these studies can be found on Pubmed.

The Endocrinology and Diabetes division of the University of California published a very comprehensive article back in July 2010 that summarizes some of the factors discussed here as well as several other things that can be considered for autoimmune thyroid conditions. This article is titled "Environmental Exposures and Autoimmune Thyroid Disease" and can be found on Pubmed with a simple Internet search. This is a definitely good read if you want to get into further nitty-gritties of the condition.

What's in your shopping cart?

Today, most of the food, or probably all, that we eat comes out of the supermarkets. We've come a long way from growing our own food or even talking to the farmer who grows our food. Food today travels an average of more than a thousand miles from farm to the table. The average kitchen no longer spends time cooking the food. Most of it is pre-made or packaged food that is simply microwaved to be cooked and eaten. The convenience of the packaged food is of course in a large part responsible for this. When making changes to the dietary pattern, it is important that the pantry stocks what you can eat. If the wrong foods are not around, the adherence with the right foods gets significantly better.

Supermarkets today spend a lot of time and money analyzing the buyer trends and making their most profitable products more easily accessible to the customers. A process that is very commonly known in the business world as business intelligence. A significant amount of money is spent by the super markets analyzing such data since easy accessibility to the products and targeted discount schemes usually result in a loyal and more frequent customer. Over a period of time, this has resulted in shaping the supermarkets the way they are today. You might've observed that as you step into the market, usually you would get directly into the aisles that stock packaged food. The analysis of buying patterns has frequently shown that if a particular item is kept more accessible, it sells better. Packaged foods usually have much better margins than fresh produce and food. So no wonder that the packaged foods are way too much easily accessible than the fresh produce. When embarking on a healthy diet pattern, you would usually want to stay on the periphery of the markets. That's where the fresh produce, meats, eggs and dairy are. These are also the things that you need to get more of.

However, we all know the convenience of packaged foods these days. Hence, when it comes to packaged foods, there are a few things that you should keep in mind.

Read the Ingredient Labels

If there would be a single biggest take away from this book for your health, it would be to start reading and understanding the nutritional and Ingredient labels on the packaged foods. This of course considering that your packaged food intake is down to bare minimum with everything that you have previously learnt in this book. We discussed a lot of diet related changes in the previous chapters and this is the place where you will be implementing those when it comes to packaged foods.

The Food and Drug Administration (FDA) provides a good starting point on their website for getting familiar with the nutrition labels on the boxes. Do note that this however applies to the Nutrition Labels. When you flip the box of your favorite packaged foods, there are several things that you would notice. First of all the Nutrition Label that specifies the Calories and certain macro components of the food such as carbohydrates, proteins, fats and other things such as Cholesterol, Vitamins some important minerals etc. Secondly, the most important part is the Ingredients Label. This is where a bunch of secrets regarding the products are hidden. As a consumer, you should definitely be concerned about the ingredient labels more than the carbohydrates, fat & protein ratios of the food. You must have realized in the earlier chapters that more than the macro nutrients, the body is more concerned about the actual ingredients when you eat something.

Here are some important considerations when reading the ingredient labels. Firstly, the ingredients are always listed in the order of their quantity in the product. The first ingredient on the label is also the most used ingredient in that product. I have seen several products that list sugar as the first ingredient and those as per this rule are definitely a problem. Now there are several packaged foods that I have seen that easily get around this rule. Whereas the first ingredient might be something different, the next few ingredients would possibly be multiple different names for sugar. Thus, sugar might still be the most used ingredient in the product but would be hiding in the guise with multiple names.

Secondly, looking at the nutritional labels, you need to be well aware of the serving size used. The values on the Nutritional Labels – the little box that mentions about the carbs, fats proteins etc – are all governed by the serving size. For a box of cereals, you may sometimes notice that the serving size might be actually half of what you would usually have in a single serving. Thus the sugars mentioned on the box is actually half of what you would be consuming in a single sitting. When comparing products, it is important to consider the serving size before you start comparing the numbers for sugars, carbs and fats.

Lastly, look at the actual ingredients itself. Do the names of the ingredients look familiar to you? A lot of processed foods these days are filled with synthetic additives. Some with complex chemical names that would take a degree in chemical engineering to understand. I do assume that all these ingredients are deemed safe for us to consume. However, I do also know that there have been instances in the past where the chemical ingredient was deemed safe to be consumed just to be found with recent research that it is not. The artificial food colors are a very good example of this. Something that is banned in European countries due to medical reason and still allowed in children's products here in the United States. Given that, although the FDA tests might be legitimate based on the current scientific knowledge, when dealing with issues such as thyroid, I think it is best to avoid those ingredients until further research specifically targeted towards the well-being of thyroid are conducted on these ingredients. I am yet to find such pervasive studies and hence the chemical compounds stay out of my food plate. If you want to know what I am talking about, just flip over a packet of bread at a regular super market and you will know exactly what I am referring to. There are several names of chemical compounds that we do not understand.

The idea here is simple. Get to know your food. Get to know what is in the food and ensure that it falls within the spectrum that we discussed in some of the earlier chapters. Does the bar of chocolate contain soy lecithin? Does the can of soup contain any form of MSG that we listed earlier? Does the bread contain high fructose corn syrup? If yes, these food no longer belong to your food plate with your new diet and lifestyle.

Research Bits
The FDA provides its guidelines on reading Nutritional Facts Labels on its website www.fda.gov.

Gluten Free

As you would have seen in the previous chapters, being gluten free is very important for thyroid Hashimoto's patients. Fortunately for us, the gluten free trend is catching up very quickly and hence the super markets are now flooded with products that are labeled gluten free. The FDA has strict guidelines for the food that is labeled gluten free. In order to label food as gluten free, the FDA mandates that the food has no more than 20 parts per million of gluten. This rule also applies to products that claim "no gluten", "free of gluten" or even "without gluten" labels. Thus being gluten free is easier than ever before here in the United States. However, even gluten free foods can have similar issues with the other products that we have earlier talked about. Hence, it is important to still ensure that you read the ingredient and nutritional labels even when purchasing gluten free foods.

Fresh Produce: Fruits & Vegetables

In the earlier chapters, we discussed why Organic and non-GMO is important in general for everyone but especially for

Hashimoto's patients. When in the supermarkets, the fresh produce is generally available on the periphery. This is where you want to be more going forward.

Organic and Non-GMO food unfortunately is not the cheapest option around when it comes to grocery shopping. So it is probably given that not all your grocery might be from the organic sources. In order to aid the organic vs non-organic decision, the Environmental Working Group (EWG) has published a list of foods that they call the "Dirty Dozen" which must be purchased organic and another list called "Clean Fifteen" of foods that are OK to be purchased non-organic. The Environmental Working Group is a non-profit organization and a leading voice when it comes to anything that impacts our environment. Pesticides of course have a huge toll on our environment which is why this list finds its way on the EWG website. In fact, if you are concerned about not just your own well-being, but also well-being of the earth and what you leave behind for your kids, you should really start considering organic wherever possible. The EWG's "Shoppers Guide to Pesticides in Produce" provides the above two lists.

| Research Bits

The Environmental Working Group provides a shoppers guide that can help you make the best choices between organic and non-organic produce. This can be found at- http://www.ewg.org/foodnews/. Or just search for EWG Shoppers Guide on the Internet.

Dairy

As we get into the animal derived products such as dairy, eggs and meat, the decisions become further complicated. The variables in these cases are not just limited to pesticides, GMO and organic. Research now shows us that the way animal is fed and treated makes a lot of difference on the nutritional aspects of animal derived products. Recent studies from the American Dairy Science Association have shown changes in fatty acid profiles of milk depending on what the cows are fed. Moreover, the processing with milk also makes a difference in how the body recognizes and processes the food. The Weston A. Price Foundation published an interesting article with micro-photography of milk with various stages of processing – raw milk, pasteurized, & homogenized. It is incredible to see that the process of homogenization literally destroys the fat globules and renders the milk indigestible. Although I do not completely advocate raw milk, science does show that grass-fed, pastured milk with minimal processing is probably the best. Organic with milk, simply means that the cows were fed an organic diet. However, the diet can still be organic grains that are not part of the cow's natural diet and hence still have the fatty acid distortions that we discussed above.

Most of the dairy today available on the store shelf is also packaged in either plastic cans or paper cans with plastic lining. It has been seen that plastic usually leeches into the food causing additional toxicity issues. If you can get your milk in old fashioned glass bottles, it reduces this concern.

Unfortunately, most of the grocery stores would not stock pasteurized, grass-fed, full fat milk in glass bottles. But that's where you can start getting closer to your food source.

Several farms are now starting to raise grass fed dairy. Natural food stores also store grass fed milk with refundable glass bottles. This obviously calls for some initial work to understand where your milk comes from. But once figured out, good milk is definitely worth it.

Research Bits

A quick internet search will reveal some interesting images of microphotography of milk at various levels of processing. The original article can be found on the Weston A. Price foundation website at www.westonaprice.org or with an internet search for "*Microphotography of Raw and Processed Milk*".

Eggs

Similar to what we discussed with milk, the way hens are raised has a significant impact on the quality of eggs. Last year we shifted from organic Grade A eggs to pasture-raised eggs. The difference in the flavors now make us never go back.

There are several terms used for the eggs today and each of them mean different.

Organic: Organic again simply means that the hens are fed organic diet. The diet can still be different from the hen's natural diet. For instance, left to their natural surroundings, the chicken would be not just eating on the pasture but also pecking smaller bugs etc. So a 100% vegetarian fed diet is fairly unnatural for the chicken.

Cage-Free: Its fairly common knowledge now how the eggs are factory farmed. Lack of movement has shown to cause several diseases for the birds which in term translates to lower quality eggs. Cage-free label ensures that the hens are out of the cages. However, it would still mean that the hens are indoor and does not make any claims about what they are fed.

Pasture-Raised: Pasture raised eggs are probably the gold standard today. This label does mean a fair amount of outdoor access for the birds. When left outdoors, the birds are able to get their natural diet. Usually, this label also accompanies Organic label which ensures that whatever other diet is provided to the chicken is organic as well.

Meat

Taking the same discussion forward for meat, similar principles apply. It has been shown that similar to humans, the animals also undergo epigenetic changes based on their diet and lifestyle. For us, when consuming the meat, this means a different nutritional profile. In 2014, FDA issued a statement confirming that arsenic used in chicken feed made its way to the meat. Hence, the specific chicken feed was taken off the market by the FDA. This goes ahead to prove the significant importance of animal feed and how it impacts us when eating the animals.

Similarly to the eggs and dairy, pasture raised or grass-fed meats are pretty much a gold standard. But again, these are not to be easily found in most of the neighborhood grocery stores. But a larger numbers of farmers are now starting to raise organic, grass-fed meats and it is possible to find a farmer nearby and source your meat in bulk. Natural foods stores also have these on their shelves now albeit at a higher price tag.

▌ Research Bits

The FDA issued their statement about retracting arsenic containing chicken feed on their website. This can be found on their website at www.fda.gov or with a quick Internet Search.

In summary, when making grocery purchases, it is important to read labels – not just the nutritional information but down to the specific ingredients. Marketing claims by the food manufacturers are aimed at selling foods and the foods might not be always what the marketing claims claim they are. Understanding the ingredients tells us a better story about the foods we eat. Getting back in touch with growing our food, either growing our own or getting back in touch with the farmer is also a great way to get to know what we eat.

Sleep

A good quality sleep at night is one of the key things that can be done to help the body recover from the day to day stress that the body experiences. Human bodies are controlled by an intricate inter-balance of different processes that are governed by our biological clocks. People studying sleep call this clock – the circadian rhythm. Before just a 100 years ago, this circadian rhythm for our body was controlled by the day and night cycles as well as the seasonal cycles. As you can imagine, the advent of the electric bulb and air-conditioned homes have thrown this disturbed this rhythm. 100 years is not a significant time for the human genome to adapt to sudden extension of the day time and a perennial summer without any temperature drops during the night – all thanks to the artificial lighting and the air conditioning. This imbalance is what starts disrupting our delicate hormonal balance. As the cascading fault correction mechanisms trigger within the body, over a period of time, the smaller incremental hormonal imbalances shift towards a major downward spiral which is when we typically start running into the "diseases of the civilization". The seeds for your thyroid condition or diabetes or cardiovascular diseases have germinated years before you can even get diagnosed by the lab tests today.

There are several sleep studies done that link the disruptions of the circadian rhythms to auto-immune diseases as well as several others. Earlier in the book, I already quoted one such study done by the National Sleep Foundation finding correlations of a higher risk for multiple sclerosis with shift work done in the teens. Here are a few more that you can look at –

▌Research Bits

Shift Work in Teens Linked to Increased Multiple Sclerosis Risk: The National Sleep Foundation discusses the link between disturbances of circadian rhythms and auto-immunity with this article at (http://sleepfoundation.org/)[3]

Here is quick snap shot of some of the very common things that impact the sleep quality. This again is not a very comprehensive list but a good starting point for a lot of us. I have also seen that the individual tolerances for the triggers vary as well so you would want to experiment with what works best for your own body. For instance, I can tolerate more coffee 4 hours before bed-time than what my husband can without impacting the sleep quality.

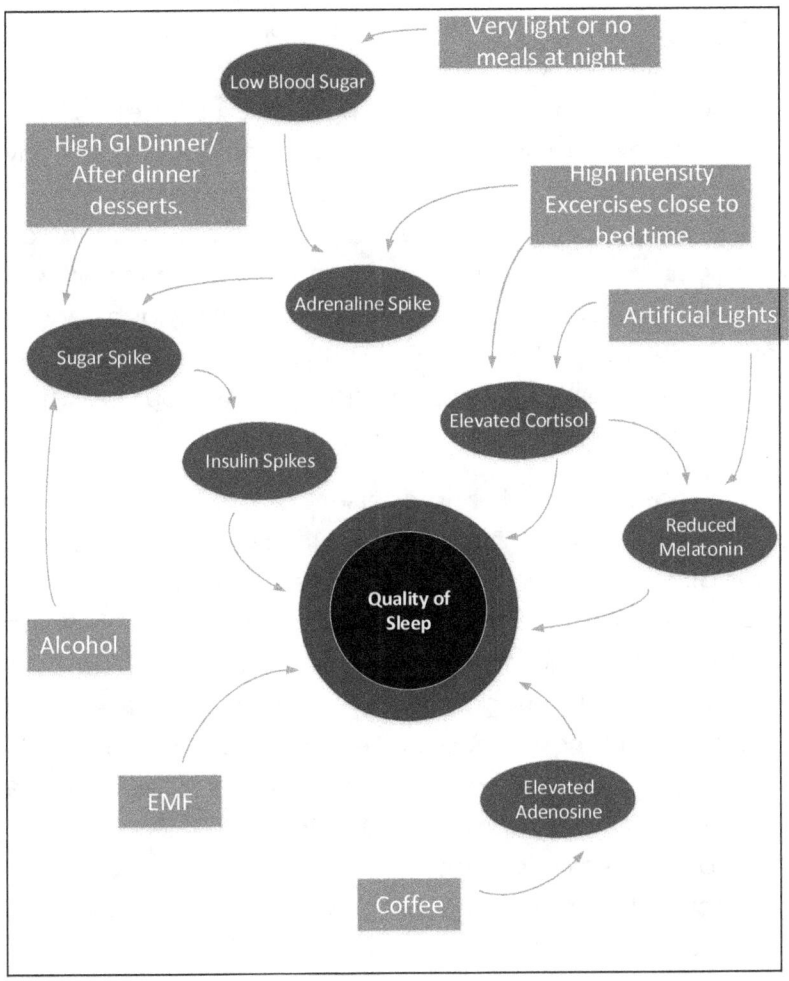

The circadian rhythms & the quality of sleep depend on some key hormones within the body – namely Melatonin, Insulin, Adrenaline & Cortisol. For a better understanding and controlling the factors essential for good sleep, it would benefit to get a quick glance at what are the various functions these hormones are responsible for. However, as we explore what these hormones do, it is important to note that the context in which these hormones operate is not a modern life-style with computer and TV screens, the work spilling into the family time, sending work emails before bed-time and everything else that we are familiar with on any given evening. The artificial lighting, TV and computers are not even a century old. Hardly a blink of an eye when you consider that the human body has not had much significant changes since last million years. The hormonal machinery still obeys the laws of our hunter gatherer ancestors as they would've lived thousands of years ago – without the latest TV series to wind down in the evening.

At a basic level, the processes within our body are metabolic. They consume energy to perform the required operations. Depending on the operations that they do, these get further categorized as either anabolic – building up things, or catabolic – tearing down things. The hormones follow a similar categorization. The thyroid hormone is a metabolic hormone since it essentially "activates" the cells to use the energy for whatever processes it is needed. The anabolic hormones promote growth within the body and catabolic hormones promote breaking down of complex molecules into much simpler ones – usually for expending energy.

Melatonin

Melatonin is more of a neuro-chemical than a hormone. But its basic understanding is crucial to understand our sleep patterns. Melatonin is our sleep inducing chemical. It's the lullaby for the brain. As the day winds down, the body starts producing melatonin. The release of this hormone as you might guess is not triggered by the Swiss clock but by changes in the ambient light and temperatures as the sun goes down. If you are continuously exposed to the sun throughout the day, before the sun down, the body starts a trickle of melatonin release. As the evening progresses to night, this trickle accumulates enough melatonin in our body to actually induce a sound sleep. That's really why you feel like falling asleep at night. This is usually inversely correlated with the Cortisol (stress hormone).

Cortisol

The Cortisol is the wakefulness hormone of the body. It is one of the anabolic hormones with responsibility to provide a burst of energy much needed in stressful situations. Not surprising that it is also known as the stress hormone. The feeling of being awake after a sound night sleep is where cortisol starts its day. Again controlled in most part by the day and night cycles, the body usually gets a shot of Cortisol with the first light of the day. Cortisol is inversely correlated with melatonin for exact same reason. Also, during stressful situations, it does not help much if you are already sleepy. You might've noticed that a stressful situation just before bed-time would not allow you to fall asleep as quickly. Now you know why. There are several other factors that can include a Cortisol burst – such as intense exercise or a stressful meeting at work. In fact, any physically or mentally stressful situation would involve Cortisol since those are the times when the body needs immediate energy to deal with the situation. Cortisol essentially works by starting to break down more complex molecular structures in the body to simpler ones such as glucose that can be used for immediate energy burn,

Insulin

With the Type 2 Diabetes rates at epidemic levels, this one of course needs no introduction. But at the same time, it needs a lot more focus since this is probably the most misunderstood amongst the hormones that are talking about. Insulin is an anabolic hormones (helps in building things). The primary function of the Insulin is of course to manage the levels of glucose in the bloodstream. For most of us, glucose is a primary fuel that our body burns. When the food is digested and converted to the glucose molecules, this glucose is delivered directly to all the cells in the body. Now most of are eating far too much sugar than what all the cells collectively need. Which is why we have higher levels of glucose circulating in the bloodstream. An elevated level of glucose is literally lethal to body mostly because it causes oxidative reactions within the body. Such reactions are linked to premature aging (of body and specific organs) and even cardio-vascular diseases. This is why Type 2 diabetics usually end up with one or more organ failures and disabilities later in life. As the Insulin cleans up the glucose and packs them in fat cells for future energy reserves, the individual cells keep consuming glucose for their energy needs. This in-turn creates a deficit and triggers the hunger signals for your body –thus disrupting a good night sleep. Ever wondered those mid-night cravings for ice-cream or cookie?

Adrenaline

Adrenaline is again not a new one for people familiar with the action sports. The rush of Adrenaline is what causes the athletes to push their bodies to the edge and most probably succeed. Typically known as Epinephrine in the medical literature, this hormone is again responsible for a quick burst of energy when dealing with a potentially dangerous situation. With a rush of adrenaline, the hormones instruct the body to provide it with some immediate source of fuel because the body is experiencing a dangerous, potentially life or death situation. It's basically "all hands on the deck". The response for the body is to spike up the blood glucose levels to provide the immediate energy by tapping into its "Glycogen" reserves. The glycogen are small cache of glucose that help the body in such dire energy situations. However, when we watch the night time soap or the new action thriller just before bed-time, sitting on a couch, we seldom put our bodies into this adrenaline rush. As the blood glucose levels increase with the surge of adrenaline, we are still sitting on the couch and the cells have no use for the extra energy. That's when insulin plays its part again and cleans up the excess glucose. So a false adrenaline response by watching a TV series or a movie is exactly the same as a high sugar dessert. On a lot of days, unfortunately, we do both.

Apart from the hormones playing part, things such as the electromagnetic radiations or frequencies have also found to be playing a part in disruption of sleep. The documentary evidence on this is not very conclusive but building up each day as more and more research on this goes through. For instance, some studies have seen that grounding the human body to earth during sleep reduces night time levels of cortisol to make them more aligned towards the 24 hour circadian profile. Now it might not be as easy to sleep on the earth each night, but this definitely hints towards more contact with the earth and nature to re-balance our circadian rhythms and hormone functioning.

As you can see here, in our day to day life, there are far too many things that can throw the sleep quality off track and far too often for the body to easily compensate. In our home, there are some simple strategies that we follow for a good night sleep.

- **NO Midnight snack:** Our body typically does not expect us to eat when we are sleeping except when we artificially alter the hormonal balance due to incorrect habits in the first place. For someone used to a daily refrigerator raid in the mid-night, it would probably take a few days to get used to this. But once some of the other strategies are addressed, this one would fall right in line.
- **NO after dinner desserts:** We discussed the insulin activity earlier. The desserts after the dinner directly fuel the insulin activity causing a sinusoidal wave of blood glucose spikes and drops throughout the night. This is also an important strategy in controlling the mid-night snack. Sometimes, if I feel a craving for a dessert, I now reach out to a 70% or 85% dark organic chocolate bars. They get me the taste of chocolate without the sugar spikes and with some good benefits of the cocoa flavonoids.
- **Reduced Carbs during dinner:** So the dinners are no longer just pasta and sauce or fried rice. It has to have a significant serving or vegetables, meat or vegetable protein and a generous addition of saturated fats – mostly in form of butter and ghee.

For those of you who are concerned about the saturated fat intake developing a risk of heart diseases, there is a growing body of evidence that the heart diseases are not being caused by the saturated fats, but due to the sugar that we consume. This of course if outside the scope of this book. I would recommend reading "Cholesterol Clarity" by Jimmy Moore & Dr. Eric Westman to understand this more.

- **NO work emails at least 30 minutes before bedtime:** As much as work is important, it can always wait. A degraded sleep quality means you would anyways not have a 100% mental focus the next day. So why degrade your input at work for the whole day when you can avoid it by just not responding to emails for 30 mins or 1 hr before bedtime? Artificial lighting and computer screens simulate day time for our body and hence induce cortisol spikes. This in-turn turns down melatonin that would otherwise help us sleep.

- **NO TV at least an hour before bedtime:** Most of the days, we do not even switch the TV. Probably the most we would do on a lot of days is when my kid gets to watch her 30 minute turn for the TV. A TV screen, similar to the computer screen induces a cortisol response, lowering the melatonin and putting your body off-track on the natural sleep schedule.

- **No Coffee or Alcohol at least 2-3 hours before bedtime:** This again is probably a no-brainer for a lot of us. Almost everyone knows that coffee disrupts sleep. Alcohol sometimes tends to make us sleep quicker. But the sleep is much lighter and breaks far more frequently.

- **No Alarm clocks:** The alarm clocks as another very common cortisol triggers. Although it still triggers it in the morning, when you do need it, it does disrupt the body from some of its precious sleep. The lost sleep accumulates over the period of time resulting in deeper hormonal issues. It is really a myth that the body needs just 7 hours of sleep each day. In fact, each of us is wired differently and would need different amounts of sleep. I usually like to take the case of pre-industrial world sleep patterns simply due to the fact that that's how our bodies are still wired up. A century of artificial lighting and work deadlines are not enough to change our wiring. Even here in the northeast parts of the US, the actual night time in the winters – from sundown to sunrise is almost 14 hours. Considering that we spend some time around the fire after the dark and getting up before sunrise, we would still be looking for at least 10-12 hours of sleep. In summer time, obeying the seasonal cycles, as the actual darkness itself was around 8-9 hours, the sleep patterns would change to reflect that. Knowing that we are not turning back from the artificial lighting, it is at least required to understand the amount of sleep our individual bodies require.

The appropriate amount of sleep needed by our bodies need to be tested out for ourselves. A week long experiment is good enough to start understanding where our sleep patterns should lie. Let's assume that you need to wake up by 6 am to be on schedule. Start by establishing a sleep time of 8 hours – so sleep at 10 PM – and see if you can wake up at 6 am without an alarm clock. If not, change the bed time accordingly. Do note however, that knowing how important it is for us to be at our workplaces each day, I would recommend doing this experiment after you are at least 3-6 months into other diet and lifestyle practices discussed in this book. Otherwise, the fluctuating thyroid levels can have a tendency for you to be in bed much longer than what your body actually needs – simply because the thyroid levels are not optimal.

Stress Management

During our discussion with sleep, we talked about the Cortisol or the stress hormone. If you are directly reading this chapter, I would highly recommend getting a basic understanding of Cortisol and its impact by reading the Sleep chapter.

Stress today is almost everywhere. Some of it is in recognizable form – work, family or financials being some of the most common forms. In other cases, it can be a bit more subtle for the body – internal body stressors such as parasite infections, food sensitivities or exposure to environmental toxins such as smoke, vehicle emissions, plastic, pesticides and a lot more things that we might not be able to put a finger on. In a nutshell, I guess we all agree that we stay in a much more stressful world than most of our ancestors from near or distant past. Hence, managing the stress is of course very critical today.

We have seen earlier that stress directly impacts the Cortisol hormone and affects sleep quality. But that's a simpler correlation to follow. Chronic stress – the case where the body gets exposed to stress (high or low grade) continuously over a period of time is what is a problem for most of us.

In the earlier chapter about sleep, we discussed how our hormones are still wired the old way. The stress hormone is no different. Stress in our body is meant to be quick and intense. Prolonged periods of stress as we undergo today, would've been fairly unknown for our distant past ancestors. Which is why the stress response mechanisms do not completely understand the low grade continuous stress. It responds to stress in the same way as it would have done some thousand years ago. Remember that just a few generations of industrialization are not sufficient enough to rewire our hormonal mechanisms and genetic expressions. These changes take thousands of years. We are moving too fast for our genes to adapt.

Typically, in a stressful situation, you would need a laser focused attention from the brain and ability to engage the muscles in the body at their full potential. In a natural circumstance, low grade stress for a longer time would usually be due to some infection or food borne illnesses. The body's natural response in such cases would be induce lethargy to promote rest and quick recovery. It's probably due to this response that the body responds by suppressing the thyroid function in event of chronic stress. Several recent research studies have found the stress on adrenaline gland or elevated levels of stress related inflammatory markers such as Interleukin-1 to be related to suppressing of the thyroid hormone. In other words, the chronic stress has a direct impact pushing you further into hypothyroidism.

A typical stress response due to elevated cortisol, as we saw earlier is also to raise the blood glucose levels. This allows the body to be alert, take immediate actions as it might expect in stressful situations. Since chronic stress continues with the same response, the body very frequently enters into a catabolic state and starts to tear down the muscle glycogen stores and in some cases also the muscles itself to start providing the glucose. Unlike the good old days, most of the stressors that we get today do not require any physical action from our body. Which is why the glucose simply stays there in the bloodstream. As the levels of glucose get higher and higher with constant stress and no action, the insulin has to kick-off to clean-up the excess glucose from the bloodstream. In effect, the chronic stress leads to a cascade of hormonal chain-reaction that would be otherwise totally unexpected and even unnecessary for the body.

The hormones in the body can be thought of as tools. Using more of them very frequently makes the body "in-sensitive" to the hormones. Thus the chain of chronic stress now starts extending to blood glucose imbalances in form of insulin resistance. Or in common terms – Type II Diabetes.

We already discussed in one of the earlier chapters how Type II Diabetes has been found to have high correlations with thyroid disorders. In essence, chronic stress is causing a double whammy on the thyroid. Not just suppressing it directly, but also possibly being suppressed due to blood glucose imbalances.

▍Research Bits

Low stress response inhibits TSH release: The 1987 study from University of Texas titled "**Central action of interleukin-1 in altering the release of TSH, growth hormone, and prolactin in the male rat**" discusses how low levels of Interluekin-1 not just stimulates growth hormone but also inhibits TSH. Another 1995 study from Tokyo titled "**Role of**

---

interleukin-1 in stress responses. A putative neurotransmitter." discusses how Interluekin-1 is involved in stress responses. When considering both these studies in conjunction with each other, we can very easily see that low level stressors negatively impact thyroid functioning.

Another 2007 study from John Hopkins School of Medicine titled "**Chemokine orchestration of autoimmune thyroiditis.**" Discusses how stress responses can decrease the sensitivity of thyroid receptors on the cells.

Another 1994 study from Italy titled "**Relationship of the increased serum interleukin-6 concentration to changes of thyroid function in nonthyroidal illness.**" Discusses how stress responses can cause low levels of T3.

All these studies can be searched for on pubmed.

With such compelling evidences of stress working against thyroid, managing stress is a critical part of thyroid management. Several stress management strategies are discussed below. But stress management is of course not contained to the strategies discussed in this book. Different branches of study discuss different mechanisms for stress management. Starting with commonly known strategies such as meditation, mindful breathing to more scientific strategies such as nutritional and supplemental support to even others such as career management, time management and much more. Let's look into some of the most potent or even the common strategies for stress management.

Meditation

Meditation perhaps is the most commonly discussed strategy for stress management. Mainstream medical science is starting to embrace this age old concept by formal studies. The Annals of Behavioral Medicine published a study in November 2014 about how meditation helped reduce cortisol levels and significantly improve the subjective quality of life of the patients. During the study, people reported lower stress levels, improved sleep, reduced symptom severity as well as reduced pain. This of course is a significant discovery in terms of how meditation helps not just calm the mind, but also help reduce the physical symptoms of the condition itself. More research is definitely warranted in this area as science starts to explore the mind-body connection. Many cultures have thoroughly explored the mind body connection. Sometimes with the rituals, other times with mindful meditation practices, still other times by emphasizing the connection with practices such as fasting etc. It is absolutely fascinating to see the science now starting to bridge the gap with better understanding of these practices. The study from Louisville School of Medicine discussed above is hence a key milestone in that respect.

The practice of meditation is perhaps not as complex as it is deemed by the most. Meditation basically refers to mindfulness or a state of hyper-awareness that has various levels of achievement. The basic state of meditation can be achieved by simply calming the responses and regulated breathing. Much more complex states of meditation allow the mind to explore the inner calmness in even completely chaotic outdoors. The first step towards a more mindful and peaceful state of mind is simply to regulate the breathing. It is common for the mind to be distracted with random thoughts, to-do lists and several other emotions when trying to focus. In order to get the mind on a single track, it is recommended to simply focus on breathing. Be aware of each breath. Focus on each breath. When a conscious focus is attempted on the breathe-ins and breathe-outs, it is fairly easy to start reducing the clutter of thoughts. As we get more and more into the practice of focusing on the breaths, we start to identify how the body responds each time we breathe in or breathe out as well as the time between the breaths. That is the state where we start to become hyper aware. Breathing is the fundamental element of life. When there is a focused effort on breathing, it starts to become more efficient. More efficient breathing also means much better oxygen delivery to the individual cells. That's probably one of the physiological reasons why mindful meditation for just 15 minutes each day freshens you up. Subsequent stages of meditation follow as we become more and more aware of the breaths and our existence in between each of those breaths. But this itself is a good start to meditation and can yield substantial benefits if followed regularly.

As we embark on the meditation journey, it is important to start with minimal distractions in possibly calm surroundings. This makes the "onboarding" process much simpler. Switch off the cell phone, get a soothing scent like lavender to aid the relaxation. Get into loose fitting clothing that does not restrict any range of motion. In other words, take care of all the common distractions that can impede your progress towards a calm thoughtless mind. Television is perhaps the most common way of breaking in and letting your mind race with new thoughts. Its best avoided before starting to meditate. When I first started getting into meditation, I realized that when everything was quite, the wall clock in my bedroom distracted me each second. If that is the case with you, or if you would now start noticing it just because it is mentioned here, get rid of the wall clock for the first few days.

Just as we are taking care of external distractions, there are several body responses that can also cause internal distractions. A rush of adrenaline or a sugar-high can cause the mind to race, thus making it difficult to rein in the mind and focus. Alcohol & Caffeine is known to cause similar behaviors in the body. On a more subtle level, the process of digestion itself requires a significant effort on the body and also causes distractions. You might've seen that it is difficult to focus immediately after a heavy meal. Well that's the digestion playing its role. Removing some of these common internal distractors are best for enhancing the meditation experience. Ensure that you do not consume alcohol, caffeine, high sugar foods or heavy meals at least 4 hours before you get down to meditate.

Essential oils such as lavender also help calm the senses and aid in the process of learning to meditate. We will explore the role of those later in this chapter as well. Soothing aroma and sounds simply help further get us into the zone. However, when using relaxing sounds, if you are tuning into music or some rhythmic acoustics, you would very soon realize that the mind wants to catch on to that and get distracted again. Sounds of nature such as bird chirps, ocean waves or wind is perhaps the best suited. Looking back at our evolutionary tracks, these are the sounds that we have evolved with. The bio-phony is what helps us get back to the roots.

Another way to remove distractions is to setup our own focal point. The visual sensory input usually floods our brain with large amount of data and makes it harder to concentrate on a specific visual input. This is where something like a chant comes handy. Several ancient cultures have perfected the art of meditating by developing their own chants. A chant is simply a word or a statement that you say over and over with each breath. The fact that you are trying to focus on the breathing and chanting at the same time, makes it easier for the brain to focus on these two activities leaving out all the other sensory inputs. A chant again should be something that relaxes your mind and does not require you to think much about it. For instance, a "Go Yankees" is probably not the most appropriate chant since it can very easily raise the adrenaline levels and pull your thoughts into the game. Most cultures usually associate chants with something divine. It is much easier to calm the mind by offloading our worries of the world to something more powerful or supernatural.

In summary, get a nice conducive environment, get rid of internal and external distractors, hone in on a soothing chant, close the eyes and focus on the breathing. That's a great way to start meditating!

There isn't an easy way to get better at calming the mind and meditating. The trick is to keep doing it each day with a routine as regular as brushing the teeth. Early morning is perhaps the best time to meditate. Especially right when we get up and the mind is yet to be pre-occupied with a lot of thoughts. If you have a luxury of being on a country side, try stepping out to meditate or get to a park. If morning perhaps is not a best time, choose a time when you want to totally unwind from the work stress. Whatever your time and place be, make a routine and stick to it!

| Research Bits

A November 2014 study from University of Louisville, Kentucky looked into the effect of meditation on conditions like fibromyalgia. They saw reduced stress, better sleep and reduced symptom severity. The study is titled "**Mindfulness Meditation Alleviates Fibromyalgia Symptoms in Women: Results of a Randomized Clinical Trial**".

All these studies can be searched for on pubmed.

Getting back in nature

Back in the 1980s, the Forest Agency of Japan proposed that people could use forests for naturally healing stress. This concept, known as *Shinrin Yoku* revolved around simply taking relaxing walks in the forest. Following that several Japanese researchers have successfully proven this with various studies around Shinrin Yoku. Shinrin Yoku encourages its participants to not just take a stroll in the park but to really engage all the five senses during the forest walk. Research has found Shinrin Yoku to be extremely relaxing experience. Similar studies performed in Europe have also found extensive correlations for stress reduction with easy access to parks and green spaces. Perhaps that is also the reason why colder places in the northern hemisphere tend to have higher incidents of depression.

From an evolutionary perspective, it is said that our bodies are tuned for last several million years to the sounds and frequencies of nature. That is possibly also the reason why our bodies respond to the frequencies, smell, sights and sounds of nature in such a healing way. Some Alternate Medicine doctors work with a concept of "Earthing" for healing their patients. We discussed this very briefly when we talked about sleep, but research has found that when the human body is in contact with the earth (ground), it has a significant positive impact on stress and circadian rhythms of the body.

Perhaps these are some of the reasons why being back in nature is one of the simplest ways to reduce stress. With the stress and engagement of day to day life, it is quite easy to forget our association with nature. It took us fairly long time to realize this missing component. But this year, the spring, summer & fall was filled with hiking, kayaking trips, beach outings or even just evenings in the park spread throughout the week. Preserving the National Parks is probably one of the best decisions the United States has made in this respect. I've been to over 20 different states thus far and realized that wherever you stay, a State Park or a National Park is never very far away. Most of the lakes and rivers have some activities such as fishing, swimming or boating (kayaking / canoeing). Community parks are usually spread across each town and city and are very easily accessible. A quick internet search can reveal a lot of avenues around you that can help you get back in touch with nature.

▍Research Bits

Shinrin Yoku has been widely studied in Japan. These studies are available on PubMed by searching for **Shinrin Yoku.**

A 2010 study in Scandinavian Journal of Public Health titled **"Health promoting outdoor environments-associations between green space, and health, health-related quality of life and stress based on a Danish national representative survey"** discusses the association between green spaces and health related quality of life. Another similar study from Finland titled **"Favorite green, waterside and urban environments, restorative experiences and perceived health in Finland"** finds similar results.

A 2013 study in International Journal of Nursing Practice titled **"Effects of Aromatherapy in relieving symptoms related to job stress amongst nurses"** discusses the use of aromatherapy to successfully handle workplace related stress.

All these studies can be searched for on pubmed.

Herbs and Scents

Several times during the course of this book, we talked about the evolutionary aspects that help set the dials within our body. Over the course of the evolution, several cultures have found and perfected the use of herbs and scents for their healing properties. The medical science of Ayurveda from ancient India is completely based on such practices. It seems this tribal knowledge was lost somewhere in the chronology and we are now re-discovering it.

Taking the baseline of Ayurveda, several studies are now being conducted to understand the impact of these herbs. A lot of these also correspond to how the herbs can help deal with stress. For instance, the holy basil plant (also known as *Tulasi*) is treated with utmost respect in India. In the good old days, each house would have at least one holy basil right outside the doorstep. The holy basil is thought to help purify the air. When eaten raw, its leaves are known to purify the blood. Studies are now also showing that the holy basil plant also helps significantly reduce stress.

Similarly the flowers of lavender are long known for their abilities to resist insects and provide a soothing smell. The studies now focusing on lavender oil aromatherapy observe that it also helps manage stress. For me, this is also one of the best sleep hacks that I would use after a long stressful day. A few drops of Lavender essential oil help calm the mind and sleep peacefully.

We discussed about Ashwagandha earlier in some of the chapters concerning the core thyroid function. This herb has also been seen to reduce stress in several studies.

Although these herbs are not known to have any detrimental side effects, it is advised to consult a medical professional who understands these herbs.

Binaural Beats

Another alternative medicine concept related to stress management is the Binaural Beats. Binaural beats work by presenting slightly different frequencies of sounds to each ears. When listened together, these kind of sounds have been seen to greatly benefit the brain function and aid sleep, relaxation & even meditation.

There are several apps available on the phone today that make binaural beats easily accessible. This might be a great place to start for managing stress levels.

Exercise & Movement

As the diet and stress levels get taken care of, the next thing to look at of course is the exercise as well as the movement in general. Exercise or rather continuous movement has shown to have significant impact on not just the overall well-being but the hormonal state as well. Not to say that one can exist without the other. Optimum health is a reflection of a good hormonal balance and vice versa. I guess in the culture that we are today, each one of us definitely understands the importance of exercise. We all know that we sit too much. Some of us spend hours on the treadmill, many of us keep making the resolutions to hit the treadmill. Our days are usually packed with long list of to-dos and exercise often takes a back seat.

So let's get to the meat of the question first – Do we really need to spend hours on the treadmill or in the gym to get to a better hormonal state? The answer of course if a big NO.

To understand how exercise impacts our hormones, lets again start looking at how our hormones were trained in the first place. During the chapter on sleep we saw that our genes and the hormones have been tuned to behave in exactly the same way as they did over tens of thousands of years ago. The recent pace of changes in our lifestyle has been too rapid for our mechanisms in the body to adapt. Having said that, let's look at this from our evolutionary lens again. Humans evolved as hunter gatherers for most part of the past. Looking at a typical day back then, we were probably on the move for most part of the day. There was not really a specific time of the day when we would get to the gym and perform body movements. Movement in essence was scattered throughout the day in various forms and not restricted to a single time within the day. Movement was also of different types and intensities depending on the situations. Our genes and hormonal responses have been structured around this frequent movement with varied intensity. For a good hormonal balance, it is required that we follow a same frequent movement patterns throughout the day. Things like taking frequent walk-breaks, doing dynamic stretches, engaging in play or other similar activities or probably the most common advice provided – walking more frequently. Admittedly, this is not going to give you the toned biceps and the six-packs. But it will surely start balancing out hormonal responses within the body.

Movement has an impact on the overall hormone profile and the cycles. Adequate movement throughout the day ensures a good blood glucose response, a more well-defined circadian rhythm and overall wellness. Although this would not directly impact the thyroid hormone, a lot of these peripheral benefits go a long way in stabilizing the thyroid hormone responses in the longer term.

There are various ways in which I try to incorporate physical movement within the daily routine. Perhaps the most commonly talked about is to walk frequently. Parking farther away from the store or office is perhaps one of the most commonly discussed tricks but at the same time least commonly used. I try to take it a step further and also use the staircase. My husband works in one of the tall buildings in downtown New York and his way of incorporating more movement is to climb up 15 flights of stairs once every week – or take the stairs at the subway station rather than escalators. But more walking does not always have to be that intense. It can start as simply as taking more 5 mins walk breaks. Get up from your seat every 45-60 mins and take a quick 5 minute walk. Probably mix that walk with some dynamic stretching. Some people I know simply add a reminder on their calendar to get up and move.

If the office allows, get a standing workstation. Standing workstations are a great way to keep the body moving without actually leaving the desk. These workstations allow you to stand and work. Once standing, it becomes fairly easy to incorporate stretches, ankle rotations and some other really basic movements while still being at your desk.

At home, some basic, inexpensive tools like medicine balls or pull-ups bar in the doorway allow adding some quick bursts of movements without compromising a lot on time. Body weight exercises of course do not need any special tools and can be done really quickly anywhere. When quick movements such as these become part of the daily lives, the question is more of doing them casually (of course with a good form) and scattering them across the day rather than earmarking 1-2 hours for exercise and keep kicking yourself when you cannot make it.

There is also a lot of innovation that can be put in with the movements. The MovNat program is a great example of this. The MovNat program is a physical fitness and education system that is based on the full range of human motion. Most of this range is usually untapped due to the constraints of our modern world. MovNat works on the principle of embedded these natural movements in the day to day life rather than a typical gym workout. Parkour or free-running, although it looks very challenging, at a basic level works on similar principles of natural and innovative movement. By innovating with movements, you will be quickly surprised at how much movement and exercise you can embed within your existing workday. Climbing stairs is probably a mundane task. Sometimes even looked upon as a tiring task at the end of the day. But try giving it a twist of innovation and it can very easily break up a lot of tension that has built up in the muscles throughout the day. Instead of typical stair climbing, try climbing it on hands and feet – on all four like a monkey. Or use your hands to propel the jump similar to that in the parkour videos. You will be surprised at how much a slight variation in this monotonous movement can help alleviate stress and rejuvenate from the day.

Movement can also be easily embedded within the family time if it becomes an integral part of what you do as a family. For instance, we will very often participate in kid's games such as tag or freeze tag. My kid's friends not just love it, but they actually think it is cool. Mundane chores like climbing stairs is made more innovative with parkour style climbs. Every morning, climbing down the stairs is a game with my husband and my daughter – she comes up with different ways of climbing down and we have to match that. Every so often she would want us to sit and climb down the stairs. A quick hang on the pull-ups bar in the door-way in a favorite pass-time each time we go under it. Movement when combined with the family time is not a drag. It actually becomes a fun thing. The next step to making it more interesting is gamification. Make a game out of it. Challenge your own limits. In the privacy of your own mind, set records and break them.

For most of the people in the gym, exercise is a set of rigid, repetitive movements. More often than not, the typical exercises are exploring only a fraction of the possible body movements. Incorporating movement in everyday life allows us to be more creative and innovative with the movements. Thus helping explore a wide range of motions that is otherwise untapped.

Experimenting with novelty skills further pushes the body into developing a wide range of motion, strength and sense of balance. All of which are very critical to the overall stability of health. Our winter weekends are usually spent at indoor rock climbing gyms or indoor trampoline parks or learning new activities such as skiing or skating or snowboarding. Spring, summer and fall are of course great times to be outdoors. We try to spend almost every evening doing some outdoor activity. Slacklining is a great activity to develop amazing balance while having a great time with kids – equally good for a group of adults. Dancing is a great way to not just incorporate a variety of movements but it also acts as a great stress buster.

As kids, we used to play an array of different games on the street. When I look at the kids today, I see that they miss out on so much fun that can be had by incorporating such playful movements within their day. Experimenting with newer things that keep challenging your range of motion is probably the best way to keep the body physically active and in a hormonally balanced state. In her book "Move your DNA", bio-mechanist Katy Bowman emphasizes on the

133

importance of overall movement that explores a variety of ranges of motion rather than the repetitive rigid sets of motions in typical exercise sessions. She attributes that to the overall wellness.

What about Cardio & High Intensity trainings?

Cardio is perhaps the first image that comes to most people's minds when they think exercise. Endless hours on the treadmill or the elliptical to "burn off the fat". You might've noticed that throughout our discussion about exercise, we never really talked about the treadmills, well almost never. Except for the statement where we mentioned that it is NOT the way to go.

So is it that so many people have really got it all wrong when it comes to exercise? If I am to talk about exercise and its impact on the hormones – yes. The runners on the treadmills do not have it right. Especially when they are running endless hours on the treadmill with the attempt to increase the heart rate in the aerobic range. There are multiple ways of increasing heart rate with exercise. For people suffering from thyroid disorders, cardio is probably one of the worst.

Exercise, in fact of any kind leads to elevation of cortisol as a natural stress response on the body. However, this kind of stress response wanes off quickly after the exercise and in fact makes the body ore adept towards handling stress. Chronic exercise such as long treadmill runs or marathons are again have a cortisol response – but in this case, much more sustained. Similar to the chronic stress that we discussed in the earlier chapter. Looking at this again from an evolutionary standpoint, there were probably far few

134

and between events when our ancestors would've needed to do long runs such as marathons. In fact, the sport of marathon actually gets its name from a place in Greek with the same name. It is said that a Greek messenger – Phillippedes – ran from Marathon to Athens to deliver the news about Greek victory against Persia. Phillippedes died right after reaching and delivering the news. Now it is not known if he died due to sheer exhaustion or some other reason. But exercise science today knows well that long distance running brings in exhaustion and has a negative impact on the hormones.

Similarly, high intensity training – although it might have patterns of similarities with the ancestral movements, does have an impact on the thyroid hormones. Especially when it is performed on a regular basis without much recovery periods in between. I have seen people doing high intensity exercises on almost daily basis and then wondering why their weight keeps increasing. Well, it is no surprise. The insufficient recovery periods are chronically suppressing the thyroid hormones. As we are all very familiar with, weight gain is a classic symptom of low levels of circulating thyroid hormones.

In last decade, exercise research has demonstrated multiple times the impact of high intensity or steady state endurance on thyroid. It has been repeatedly seen that higher volumes of exercise inhibits thyroid hormones. A lot of these studies also looked at the recovery periods. The effect on thyroid starts to become "chronic" when the recovery periods between these exercise sessions are substantially less – say when you are hitting the treadmill or doing a session of tennis or rounds of cycling every single day! In other words, when dealing with hypo-thyroid related weight gain, the high volume of exercise is not helping but actually contributing to the weight gain.

Research Bits

A 2006 study in Turkey, titled **"The effect of exhaustion exercise on thyroid hormones and testosterone levels of elite athletes receiving oral zinc"** noted a significant inhibition of thyroid hormones due to exhaustion in elite wrestlers.
Another 2005 study from Turkey found a decrease in circulating T3 hormones with moderate to high intensity aerobic exercises – in this case riding a bicycle. This study is aptly titled **"Exercise intensity and its effects on thyroid hormones"**
A 2012 study from North Carolina, USA, titled **"Thyroid hormonal responses to intensive interval versus steady-state endurance exercise sessions"** looks at thyroid responses to Steady state endurance exercises and High intensity Interval trainings. This study also looks at the hormone levels post 12-hour – thus emphasizing the recovery period.
All these studies can be searched for on pubmed.

In summary, movement – and a variety of it – is definitely required to maintain a great sense of well-being and an on overall hormonal balance. This hormonal balance in turn ensures a lot of peripheral things around the thyroid well-being. However, exercise in the traditional sense is probably best avoided or done with a great thought towards recovery. The mindless hamster wheel type running on the treadmill each day is definitely a killer for the thyroid.

Thyroid Management Protocol

We looked at all the science and why it is important for us to do all the things that we discussed. Now here are some quick practical tips to get you started. First of all, I would recommend that you take a copy of this pyramid and stick it on your desk or refrigerator or someone where this stays in front of you all the time. It helps to have a regular reminder of where you want to be.

The Thyroid Management Pyramid is divided into Four Levels. The Base Level – Level 1, is a non-negotiable. This alone demonstrates a significant impact on the thyroid function. The remaining can be taken in order of precedence depending on which level they fall in. This pyramid summarizes all the things that you can do today to positively impact your thyroid condition.

Do not worry if you cannot do this all in the first attempt. Lifestyle changes are hard. But they yield results. It took me 6 months to incorporate all these changes. Even today, during winters when there is a couple of feet of snow outside, I miss on my frequent movement. But the goal here is not perfection. The goal is to strive to do more of the things that are right for your body. The goal is to get rid of the prescriptions to whatever extent possible in the safest possible way. The goal is to feel great when you wake up in the morning and have the energy to be able to enjoy the life the way you want to. Each step, no matter how small, is taking you closer to your goal.

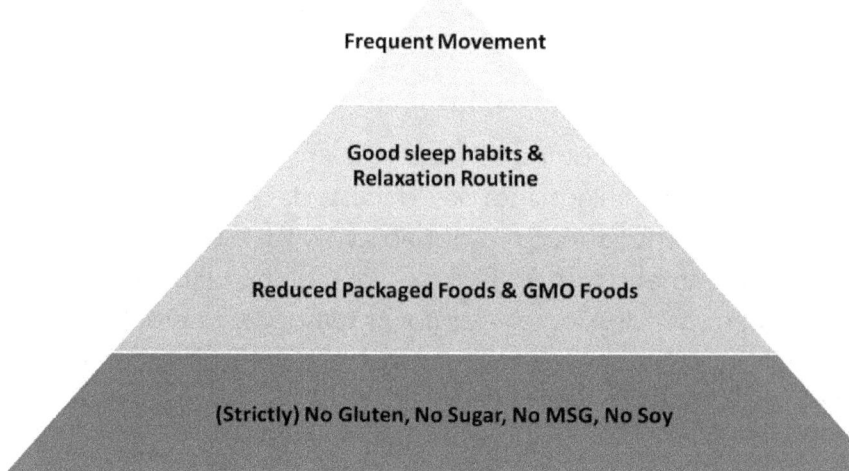

Frequent Movement

Good sleep habits & Relaxation Routine

Reduced Packaged Foods & GMO Foods

(Strictly) No Gluten, No Sugar, No MSG, No Soy

Level 1: No Gluten, No Sugar, No MSG, No Soy.

This is a non-negotiable. The chapter Re-designing the Food Plate discusses the reasons in much more details. Gluten, Soy are very common triggers for auto-immunity. From my personal experience, I have seen that when I accidentally introduce gluten even for one meal, it takes me almost 3-6 months to get back to a better state on physical being. The symptoms are usually what I used to have. What I really dread now. Sugars are not just the plain old sugar cubes here but also sugars from other sources (including the simple carbohydrate sources). My husband and I did a small experiment on a group on a social networking site. It was a

30-day sugar challenge – for a group of approximately 25 people. Eliminating all sugars caused interesting positive reactions. Most people reported weight loss, but then people also reported much better energy constantly throughout the day.

Cutting down Gluten & Soy is easier. Sugar is slightly more difficult due to the pervasiveness. Start taking it week by week with each of these. Most importantly, do not get dejected if you cannot do it in the first shot. Neither did I do this right away. It took me 3 months to get off gluten and soy. For sugar, it was over 6 months. Slowly wane off these foods and once you are out of them, stay out.

Level 2: Reduced Packaged Foods and GMO

If you might not have already realized managing the thyroid needs you to get back in the kitchen. Cook more often. The chapter "What's in your shopping cart" talks a lot about the processed foods found in most grocery stores today. Get ingredients that are found in nature – that does not include pop tarts and cheerios. Get fresh ingredients and cook them yourself. Know what you are eating. Preferably, know where your food is coming from.

A weekly trip to the farmers market not just reduces your accessibility to packaged foods but also gets you in touch with the people who are growing your food. Talk to them, get know. A large part of enjoying the food is also knowing where it came from. In the medieval Europe, each family would have their own pigs and birds. When the animal was served at the dinner table, most often they would know even its name – not just what it ate and how it lived.

Although today we might not see the little Lucy with pink ears on the table, it is important today more than any other time in history to know how the animal was raised. Get to know the farmer. Talk about their practices. In the process you will also have some of your own stories to talk about on the dining table when you sit together for a family dinner.

Level 3: Good sleep habits and relaxation routine

The Chapters about "Sleep" and "Stress Management" discuss how important it is to lower your stress and rejuvenate your body with sleep each night. Get into a practice of 5 minute meditation every day. Kick the habits of alcohol or coffee in the evening. Prepare a sleeping routine. Check-out of your work way before your bed time.

At least once or twice a week, take a stroll in the community park. Meet people outdoors. Experience being with nature. Probably nurture a hobby like gardening that will not just put you in contact with the nature but will also provide you with fresh foods. Who wants to do weekly grocery store trips anyways? You can save those trips for a walk in the park.

Level 4: Frequent Movement

Lastly, the "Exercise & Movement" chapter talks about the ideal exercise routine that research suggests for people with thyroid disorders. The best exercise really is no-exercise. But instead, having frequent, varied low intensity movements throughout the day. The household chores, a walk around the block, sitting on the floor rather than the sofa. There are multiple ways to include small sets of movements throughout the day. Be ingenious. Figure out a way to include movement in everything that you do. Sitting on a desk? Perhaps, start by small ankle rotations, small foot movements such as calf stretches. These movements are usually so subtle that your colleague sitting right next to you would not even know that you are moving. Take a quick 3-5 minutes break every 30 minutes or at least every one hour and walk around the office. Do other smaller movements such as neck rotations, wrist rotations. There is so much to include just when you are at the desk. When walking, instead of plain old walks, try skipping or doing short jumps. Give your body a variety of movements to work with.

Research Links

All the relevant links for the research mentioned in the research bits throughout the book as well as a lot of research that provided the underlying thought process and the breadcrumbs is listed here. I would encourage you to go through these links and use the knowledge when working towards your condition. The interpretation of the research is lot of times subject to the context that the research is read with. In addition to that the research conducted is often targeted to prove certain pre-existing theory which would make the setup of the research biased towards a certain output. These are very frequently the cases when the research is targeted towards a particular pharmaceutical compound and is funded by the pharmaceutical company itself. Hence, reading the research with our own context and assimilating that information to analyze how it impacts your own condition is always recommended. I would also encourage to take some of this research into your conversations with your own doctor to help clarify it further in your specific context.

There is a vast amount of scientific literature surrounding thyroid auto-immune conditions. Hence, I also argue that you do not stop with what you find in this book. Rather, use it as a Launchpad to delve further. No one understands your body better than yourself. Armed with the appropriate information and a good partnership with an open-minded doctor would allow you to take charge of your own health and drive it rather than being driven around. If we have any hopes of getting better, we need to take charge and not be convinced with an answer that squarely blames everything on genetics or lifestyle. Epigenetics has shown us that our genes can change with lifestyle changes. Lifestyle change is probably the simplest things we would be able to do today considering that it will help us get out of a future where we are dependent on medications for our basic survival.

When I started researching Hashimoto's, after some initial leads into gluten sensitivity, I literally kept asking the why & how questions each time. These acted as bread crumbs that I could follow to seek all the information that I was able to put together in this book. The information obviously is simplified here. But the research links below can take you down the rabbit hole as deep as you would want to go.

So go ahead, explore, research and get on a path to a healthy life.

1) Hypothyroidism - National Endocrine and Metabolic Diseases Information Service (NEMDIS); 2014; http://www.endocrine.niddk.nih.gov/pubs/hypothy roidism/index.aspx
2) Autoimmune thyroid diseases and coeliac disease. European Journal of Gastroenterology & Hepatology; 1998, Nov; Sategna-Guidetti C, Bruno

M, Mazza E, Carlino A, Predebon S, Tagliabue M, Brossa C.;
http://www.ncbi.nlm.nih.gov/pubmed/9872614

3) Shift Work in Teens Linked to increased Multiple Sclerosis Risk. National Sleep Foundation;
http://sleepfoundation.org/sleep-news/shift-work-teens-linked-increased-multiple-sclerosis-risk

4) Alterations in Intestinal Permeability; 2006, Oct; M C Arrieta, L Bistritz, and J B Meddings;
http://www.ncbi.nlm.nih.gov/pmc/articles/PMC1856434/

5) Bugs & us: The role of the gut in autoimmunity; Nov 2012; David Luckey, Andres Gomez, Joseph Murray, Bryan White and Veena Taneja;
http://www.ncbi.nlm.nih.gov/pmc/articles/PMC3928703/

6) New diseases derived or associated with the tight junction;
http://www.ncbi.nlm.nih.gov/pubmed/17560451

7) Bugs & Us: The role of gut in auto-immunity;
http://www.ncbi.nlm.nih.gov/pmc/articles/PMC3928703/

8) Adrenal stress suppresses t4 to t3 -
http://www.ncbi.nlm.nih.gov/pubmed/8180680

9) Chemokine orchestration of autoimmune thyroiditis;
http://www.ncbi.nlm.nih.gov/pubmed/17910527/

10) Intestinal permeability and nutritional status in developmental disorders. ;
http://www.ncbi.nlm.nih.gov/pubmed/22516881

11) Psychological stress and corticotropin-releasing hormone increase intestinal permeability in humans by a mast cell-dependent mechanism;
http://www.ncbi.nlm.nih.gov/pubmed/24153250

12) Relationship of the increased serum interleukin-6 concentration to changes of thyroid function in nonthyroidal illness; http://www.ncbi.nlm.nih.gov/pubmed/7930379

13) Reversible subclinical hypothyroidism in the presence of adrenal insufficiency; http://www.ncbi.nlm.nih.gov/pubmed/17002934

14) Chemokine orchestration of autoimmune thyroiditis

15) Circadian Rhythm and the Immune response: A Review; http://www.ncbi.nlm.nih.gov/pubmed/19241255

16) Sleep, Immunity and Circadian Clocks: A Mechanist Model; http://www.ncbi.nlm.nih.gov/pubmed/20130392

17) Sunlight and vitamin D for bone health and prevention of autoimmune diseases, cancers, and cardiovascular disease; http://www.ncbi.nlm.nih.gov/pubmed/15585788

18) Vitamin D: modulator of the immune system; http://www.ncbi.nlm.nih.gov/pubmed/20427238

19) Vitamin D toxicity redefined: vitamin K and the molecular mechanism; http://www.ncbi.nlm.nih.gov/pubmed/17145139

20) Novel role of the vitamin D receptor in maintaining the integrity of the intestinal mucosal barrier; http://www.ncbi.nlm.nih.gov/pubmed/17962355

21) Vitamin D and immunity; http://www.ncbi.nlm.nih.gov/pubmed/25580272

22) Vitamin D status and its association with adiposity and oxidative stress in schoolchildren; http://www.ncbi.nlm.nih.gov/pubmed/25102819

23) Relationship of Serum Magnesium and Vitamin D Levels in a Nationally-Representative Sample of

Iranian Adolescents: The CASPIAN-III Study; http://www.ncbi.nlm.nih.gov/pubmed/24554998/

24) The Normal TSH Reference Range: What has Changed in the last decade

25) Thyroid dysfunction in patients with diabetes: clinical implications and screening strategies;2010 July; Prince Charles Hospital; Cwm Taf Local Health Board; Merthyr Tydfil
http://www.ncbi.nlm.nih.gov/pubmed/20642711

26) Cardiovascular risk factors in children with type 1 diabetes and their relationship with the glycemic control;
http://www.ncbi.nlm.nih.gov/pubmed/16296632

27) Sugar and chromosome stability: clastogenic effects of sugars in vitamin b6-deficient cells;
http://www.plosgenetics.org/article/info%3Adoi%2F10.1371%2Fjournal.pgen.1004199

28) Thyroid gland diseases in adult patients with diabetes mellitus; Dec 2005; Vondra K1, Vrbikova J, Dvorakova K.;
http://www.ncbi.nlm.nih.gov/pubmed/16319810

29) Oral bioavailability of glyphosate: studies using two intestinal cell lines;
http://www.ncbi.nlm.nih.gov/pubmed/?term=glyphosate+intestinal+permeability

30) Glyphosate-Based Herbicides Potently Affect Cardiovascular System in Mammals: Review of the Literature;
http://www.ncbi.nlm.nih.gov/pubmed/25245870

31) FDA: How to understand and use Nutrition Facts label;http://www.fda.gov/Food/IngredientsPackagingLabeling/LabelingNutrition/ucm274593.htm#footnote

32) FDA labeling laws for "gluten free" (www.fda.gov)

33) 3-Nitro (Roxarsone) and Chicken;
http://www.fda.gov/AnimalVeterinary/SafetyHealth
/ProductSafetyInformation/ucm257540.htm

34) Microphotography of Raw and Processed Milk;
http://www.westonaprice.org/health-
topics/microphotography-of-raw-and-processed-
milk/

35) Intense sweetness surpasses cocaine reward;
http://www.ncbi.nlm.nih.gov/pubmed/17668074

36) Evidence for sugar addiction: behavioral and
neurochemical effects of intermittent, excessive
sugar intake;
http://www.ncbi.nlm.nih.gov/pubmed/17617461

37) Aspartame, low-calorie sweeteners and disease:
regulatory safety and epidemiological issues;
http://www.ncbi.nlm.nih.gov/pubmed/23891579

38) Neurobehavioral Effects of Aspartame
Consumption;
http://www.ncbi.nlm.nih.gov/pubmed/24700203

39) USDA National Organic Program;
http://www.ams.usda.gov/AMSv1.0/NOPOrganicSt
andards

40) Pesticides in mixture disrupt metabolic regulation;
http://www.ncbi.nlm.nih.gov/pubmed/24530807

41) Environmental Exposures and Autoimmune Thyroid
Disease; Jul 2010; Gregory A. Brent;
http://www.ncbi.nlm.nih.gov/pmc/articles/PMC293
5336/

42) Cognitive and biochemical effects of monosodium
glutamate and aspartame, administered
individually and in combination in male albino
mice;
http://www.ncbi.nlm.nih.gov/pubmed/24556450

43) Transplacental neurotoxic effects of monosodium glutamate on structures and functions of specific brain areas of filial mice;
http://www.ncbi.nlm.nih.gov/pubmed/8085168

44) Toxic effects of some synthetic food colorants and/or flavor additives on male rats;
http://www.ncbi.nlm.nih.gov/pubmed/22317828

45) Biochemical effect of chocolate colouring and flavouring like substances on thyroid function and protein biosynthesis;
http://www.ncbi.nlm.nih.gov/pubmed/1717848

46) Bone and Vegetable Broth;
http://www.ncbi.nlm.nih.gov/pmc/articles/PMC1975347/

47) Enhanced intestinal anastomotic healing with gelatin hydrogel incorporating basic fibroblast growth factor;
http://www.ncbi.nlm.nih.gov/pubmed/24130076

48) Traditional Bone Broth in Modern Health and Disease

49) Protective effect of Curcumin on chemotherapy-induced intestinal dysfunction;
http://www.ncbi.nlm.nih.gov/pmc/articles/PMC3816802/

50) Protective effect of curcumin against methotrexate-induced small intestinal damage in rats;
http://www.ncbi.nlm.nih.gov/pubmed/18227041

51) Are there any different effects of Bifidobacterium, Lactobacillus and Streptococcus on intestinal sensation, barrier function and intestinal immunity in PI-IBS mouse model?;
http://www.ncbi.nlm.nih.gov/pubmed/24595218

52) Prebiotics to fight diseases: reality or fiction?; http://www.ncbi.nlm.nih.gov/pubmed/23280537

53) Withania somnifera and Bauhinia purpurea in the regulation of circulating thyroid hormone concentrations in female mice; http://www.ncbi.nlm.nih.gov/pubmed/10619390

54) Changes in thyroid hormone concentrations after administration of ashwagandha root extract to adult male mice; http://www.ncbi.nlm.nih.gov/pubmed/9811169

55) The importance of selenium in Hashimoto's disease; http://www.ncbi.nlm.nih.gov/pubmed/25228521

56) Soy isoflavones interfere with thyroid hormone homeostasis in orchidectomized middle-aged rats; http://www.ncbi.nlm.nih.gov/pubmed/24793811

57) Unawareness of the effects of soy intake on the management of congenital hypothyroidism; http://www.ncbi.nlm.nih.gov/pubmed/22908106

58) Environmental Exposures and Autoimmune Thyroid Disease; http://www.ncbi.nlm.nih.gov/pmc/articles/PMC2935336/

59) Central action of interleukin-1 in altering the release of TSH, growth hormone, and prolactin in the male rat; http://www.ncbi.nlm.nih.gov/pubmed/3500324

60) Role of interleukin-1 in stress responses. A putative neurotransmitter; http://www.ncbi.nlm.nih.gov/pubmed/7598832

61) Mindfulness Meditation Alleviates Fibromyalgia Symptoms in Women: Results of a Randomized Clinical Trial; Annals of Behavioral Medicine; 2014, Nov; University of Louisville school of medicine; http://www.ncbi.nlm.nih.gov/pubmed/25425224

62) The effects of aromatherapy in relieving symptoms related to job stress among nurses;
http://www.ncbi.nlm.nih.gov/pubmed/24238073

63) Constituents of Ocimum sanctum with antistress activity;
http://www.ncbi.nlm.nih.gov/pubmed/17850106

64) The biologic effects of grounding the human body during sleep as measured by cortisol levels and subjective reporting of sleep, pain, and stress;
http://www.ncbi.nlm.nih.gov/pubmed/15650465

65) Psychological effects of forest environments on healthy adults: Shinrin-yoku (forest-air bathing, walking) as a possible method of stress reduction.
http://www.ncbi.nlm.nih.gov/pubmed/17055544

66) Psychological relaxation effect of forest therapy: results of field experiments in 19 forests in Japan involving 228 participants].
http://www.ncbi.nlm.nih.gov/pubmed/21996766

67) Favorite green, waterside and urban environments, restorative experiences and perceived health in Finland;
http://www.ncbi.nlm.nih.gov/pubmed/20176589

68) Health promoting outdoor environments-- associations between green space, and health, health-related quality of life and stress based on a Danish national representative survey.;
http://www.ncbi.nlm.nih.gov/pubmed/20413584

69) Aerobic exercises reduce T3 & fT3 levels in blood. Exercise intensity and its effects on thyroid hormones;
http://www.ncbi.nlm.nih.gov/pubmed/16380698

70) Exhaustion leads to inhibition of thyroid in wrestlers;
http://www.ncbi.nlm.nih.gov/pubmed/16648789

71) Exercise intensity and its effects on thyroid
   hormones;
   http://www.ncbi.nlm.nih.gov/pubmed/16380698
72) Thyroid hormonal responses to intensive interval
   versus steady-state endurance exercise sessions;
   http://www.ncbi.nlm.nih.gov/pubmed/22450344
73)

_____

www.ingramcontent.com/pod-product-compliance
Lightning Source LLC
Chambersburg PA
CBHW070355290526
45790CB00004B/1507